I HATE
YOGA

And Why You'll Hate to Love it Too

PAUL MCQUILLAN

NEW YORK

I HATE YOGA
And Why You'll Hate to Love it Too

Published in New York, New York, by Morgan James Publishing. Morgan James and The Entrepreneurial Publisher are trademarks of Morgan James, LLC. www.MorganJamesPublishing.com

The Morgan James Speakers Group can bring authors to your live event. For more information or to book an event visit The Morgan James Speakers Group at www.TheMorganJamesSpeakersGroup.com.

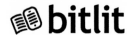

A free eBook edition is available with the purchase of this print book.

CLEARLY PRINT YOUR NAME ABOVE IN UPPER CASE

Instructions to claim your free eBook edition:
1. Download the BitLit app for Android or iOS
2. Write your name in **UPPER CASE** on the line
3. Use the BitLit app to submit a photo
4. Download your eBook to any device

ISBN 978-1-63047-412-6 paperback
ISBN 978-1-63047-414-0 eBook
ISBN 978-1-63047-413-3 hardcover
Library of Congress Control Number:
2014949060

Cover Design by:
Chris Treccani
www.3dogdesign.net

Interior Design by:
Bonnie Bushman
bonnie@caboodlegraphics.com

In an effort to support local communities, raise awareness and funds, Morgan James Publishing donates a percentage of all book sales for the life of each book to Habitat for Humanity Peninsula and Greater Williamsburg.

Get involved today, visit
www.MorganJamesBuilds.com.

I HATE YOGA

To my blood family, my yoga family
and my theatre family;
a trilogy of inspiration

CONTENTS

FOREWORD

By **Pattie Lovett-Reid**
(Chief Financial Commentator CTV News)

If you had to classify my personality, most would say I'm a type A++ individual. I'm focused, goal-oriented and I love to track my progress. Seeing immediate results is important to me—in fact, I measure a great day by how many tasks I am able to cross off my to-do list, and I subscribe to the philosophy that only the boring are bored.

I've always worked out regularly; biking, swimming and running long-distance races—partly motivated by the shock of having my father die of a heart attack at the age of 36.

A few years back, I went for my annual physical and discovered that I was in the 90th percentile—relative to my age (I'm 56)—in strength, endurance and cardio.

Flexibility? 5th percentile.

I was stunned, but I'm not sure why—not only couldn't I reach my toes, I couldn't even touch my *knees*! The prescription I took away was simple enough: You need to do yoga. Now.

There was only one problem: I *hated* yoga. My perception of yoga was that it was slow and dull. I liked activities that gave me a high and left me with a feeling of accomplishment— surely *yoga* couldn't measure up to my standards.

I needed to find a way to get excited about yoga.

A friend who knew the challenge I was now facing invited me to a Bikram yoga class. I agreed to try it, although *very* reluctantly. It was hot, long (90 minutes), and worst of all, there was no talking allowed. Can you imagine? I make a living by talking.

Yet, something very special happened in that first class: I felt strangely quiet, settled, and at peace in that room. There were no expectations of me—no judging, no competing or comparing. And it was *anything* but slow or dull. In fact, the challenge was exhilarating and the yoga enabled me to satisfy my goal of achieving more flexibility.

I hit the jackpot.

But if yoga is synonymous with balance, I still had a lot to learn. I started to become obsessive about practicing yoga, believing that if 3 or 4 times a week was good for me, 6 or 7 must be even better—for some it's fine, but in my case, it just wasn't.

I overdid it and landed in the hospital with severe dehydration and at risk of a heart attack. I was terrified that history may have a way of repeating itself.

The irony of it all was lost on me.

Fortunately, I have since found a necessary balance that enables me to benefit from yoga, which was the point all along.

Now, I love yoga. I schedule it into every week and have an innate belief that it will extend the quality of my life; I can feel it—but it's a feeling that came through the discovery that even *yoga* can be of detriment if its not molded to cater to an individual's subjective needs.

It's a love-hate relationship, which brings me to this book, *I Hate Yoga*.

First, let me say a bit about Paul.

I am fortunate to have him as my friend and yoga instructor. He is focused, driven and passionate. He wants you to give your best, but never expects you to be the best. The minute he sees your ego sabotaging your efforts, he will call you on it. His humor adds a much-needed levity to every class, and he offers a refreshing perspective on yoga that doesn't glorify the subject.

We have all faced journeys that involve both love and hate. *I Hate Yoga* takes us on one such journey—an enlightening, hysterical ride that will give you the opportunity to reflect upon how *you* feel about yoga and, ultimately, how you may just be able to benefit from it.

I love Paul's book. For an activity where you aren't allowed to speak he has a lot to say that will get you fired up and want to join in. It's fast-paced and sprinkled generously with humor as he breaks down common myths and separates them from the facts. This book is inspiring and the words are encouraging—and if you are willing to plant your tongue firmly in your cheek and not take yourself too seriously, you can embark on your own love-hate journey of self-discovery with *I Hate Yoga*.

Take it from this type A++ personality. I learned—with yoga as my guide—that it is more important to listen to yourself and to your body than it is to tick a task off your to-do list.

Yoga helped me feel like I can take on the world…one breath at a time. Now, take your own big breath, and dive in!

INTRODUCTION

"I love you and because I love you, I would sooner have you hate me for telling you the truth than adore me for telling you lies."

—Pietro Aretino

I hate yoga.

I really do. I don't state this for effect.

Being grateful for something that has given me healing, prosperity, purpose, and meaningful relationships would be the evolved disclosure here.

But it isn't. Because I hate it.

I'm too alarmingly focused on what contemporary Western society has done to yoga to find solace or understanding in the word anymore. Like many things in the Western world, yoga has been bastardized beyond recognition, to the point where saying it's an authentic form of healing would be a great disservice to the sacred origin of the word. But after all, going to McDonald's for a salad is like going to a hooker for a hug.

North America is the hooker. Yoga is the hug. Just clarifying.

So few people in North America, especially teachers of yoga and supposed "gurus," actually know what yoga really is.

I certainly don't, and I've been teaching it for nine years, but I know this: I hate it. I have to. It's the only way to love it again.

The multiplying spawn of self-righteous yoga "knowers" must be obliterated. A yoga war must ensue, and I will begin by turning the gun on myself.

Being a card-carrying member, I know what it will take to destroy such a breed. An exorcism must be performed—one that holds me and all "yoga experts" out there accountable for what we're doing.

If it seems like I'm tossing blame by starting the healing with yoga-hate, let me explain my theory for therapy.

Sometimes it's necessary to hate something in order to revive its credibility and actually benefit from it. It's not unlike the feelings many of us have experienced at the end of a nasty relationship. We hate that person—for a while, anyway. Then, after a varying amount of time passes, that feeling dissipates, the vitriol subsides, the whole experience just becomes information, and we can look at it all with some insight and clarity.

Then, if the stars align, as they should, we learn.

Only then can we proceed responsibly and progressively with regards to the subject, person, or situation that has been a tainted aspect of our history.

It's important to understand something: The first half of this book isn't about waxing poetic over the merits of yoga; pretentiousness cannot be part of the blueprint here.

It's about dismantling the pseudo-merits so that that we can uncover what's truly useful and start fresh.

Don't worry. We'll get the hate out of the way quickly enough, but it's an integral part of the path.

In the teachings of Buddhism, one is told, "If you meet the Buddha, kill the Buddha." In other words, we are always on a journey with no destination. If we ever feel like we've arrived, we didn't really get the point. To name it is to not really know it.

Let's kill yoga and all of the bullshit that has manifested around it. It's time to let it die in our blood-soaked hands on our bullet-ridden yoga mats.

We're going to do this together because here's another admission: This book isn't about me. It's about you—and what you can get from this increasingly tarnished word, "yoga," by simply stripping it of all its labels and ludicrous expectations.

And then, by practicing it.

I think I can help. As a matter of fact, I know I can.

Once we have cathartically performed our ugly yoga striptease and thrown down each garment of bogus credibility and confusion, we will then focus on watching the Yoga-Phoenix rise from the ashes.

We'll remove the bewildering fear factor surrounding yoga and explore the truth behind the practice, revealing it to be a great healer. While on this journey, we will discover that yoga is wonderfully accessible to all of us.

This will take place only after the affectations surrounding yoga have been laid bare and exposed as nothing more than a societal red herring, distracting us from the beauty of a profoundly beneficial art form.

I want *you* to be the beneficiary.

Hang on, though. This first part could get a little ugly.

PART 1

KILLING YOGA

Chapter 1

MY JOURNEY
TO YOGA-HATE

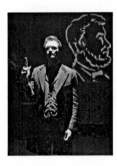

Paul McQuillan as
John Wilkes Booth
in award-winning
production of
Assassins, 2011.

"Toto, I've a feeling we're not in Kansas anymore!"
—Dorothy (*Wizard of Oz*)

I grew up in London, Ontario Canada with a lot of white people. If there was any kind of ethnic diversity in London it certainly escaped my upbringing. My growth progression was very linear:

Go to school with white people; play hockey with white people; go to Catholic church with other less-than-willing young white people; and finally, have sex for the first time at the age of sixteen—with a white person.

To enhance the white people formula even further, I'm Scottish. Most Scottish people are very white, and I'm no exception. My mother and father were born in Glasgow as were my three older siblings, but obviously feeling like I wasn't quite owning my whiteness, they raised me in London just to make sure I had the white thing down. I did. And I was good at it.

That is, until I decided to leave London at the age of eighteen for music theatre college. I went from wasp-London to a town called Oakville, just outside of Toronto, to learn how to further my potentially promising singing and acting abilities.

It was only then that my perspective changed dramatically.

It would have been like watching an old Charlie Chaplin film with no sound or color only to suddenly be thrown into an IMAX 3D movie of *The Adventures of Priscilla, Queen of the Desert!*

Gay people. Black people. Asians. Hispanics. They were everywhere.

I was sure there were no gay people in London because no one mentioned anything. Now I lived close to a city where they had parades that answered all your questions—even the ones you didn't ask.

In music theatre college, you were gay unless someone told you otherwise.

All of this is to say that my upbringing was somewhat sheltered in good ol' London, so my early years did not prepare me to paint my world with a broad stroke of cultural insight or understanding.

I was gullible, green, and ridiculously impressionable.

But regardless of our whitewashed view of the world, racism was not instilled in me simply because I wasn't exposed to other cultures. I share the belief with many that racism is learned. Luckily, it wasn't on the family curriculum.

My parents were more focused on putting food on the table than issues. For two young (somewhat poor) adults in Glasgow in the 1950s, the focus was simple: Make enough money to feed your children. That theme stayed consistent well into my early years. So, anything resembling gender-bias or racism would have taken a backseat for my parents around the same time that Rosa Parks refused to take hers.

This admission will serve its purpose later, given my current fascination with the multicultural environment I currently enjoy in Toronto.

In college I was stripped of my cultural naiveté and, with it, most of my talent—at least for a while.

The culture changes were actually quite refreshing. My difficulties arose from being shocked into submission by the systematic decimation of my confidence, instinct, and natural ability by almost every instructor in the school. One new teacher did his best to steer me in the right direction, but ultimately fell prey to the peer-induced drama surrounding him as well.

Despite winning the award for "most promising first year student," I was drowning in a sea of insecurity, which was radiating toxically from the teachers around me—many failed or semi-successful actors or singers with personal agendas so aggressively Machiavellian, they would make Napoleon look like Richard Simmons.

Sadly, this energy was contagious, and there was no antidote.

It wasn't until I left college after three years that I rediscovered my gifts, embraced their uniqueness, and quickly landed a Broadway show called *The Buddy Holly Story*. It was my first big show, followed by many more and a thirty-year career in music theatre which would include two Dora Mavor Moore Award nominations (Toronto's Tony Awards, minus the hype) for Best Actor in a Musical.

But it's important to point out that I had to unlearn what I was taught at school—which in retrospect did more harm than good—and return to something that carried no motive or agenda: my instincts.

I had to embrace my essence as opposed to fight it. It certainly wasn't going to come to fruition through the projected angst of angry singing instructors or self-righteous drama dudes.

I had to feel safe. Only then could I thrive.

Later on, yoga would take a large role in maximizing this feeling of safety, propelling me into a world of confidence that I only could have dreamed of in college.

And then, sneakily and with less warning, yoga—with its own suspect devices—would also begin to strip me of the same joy it had doled out so generously.

But let's not go there yet. A little more of my story first …

Confidence in my ability as a performer landed me many great roles throughout the years including a two-year stint as Corny Collins in the hit musical *Hairspray,* which, interestingly enough, told the story of a young girl in '60s Baltimore transcending a landscape of racism, discrimination, and segregation to unearth her natural talent to the world—a more dramatic telling of what might have gone on in my hometown of London if any black people actually lived there.

While *Hairspray* didn't parallel my upbringing at all, it may have resonated with me so deeply because of the guilt I felt for not knowing such adversity was taking place around me in other parts of the world while I grew up. I was making up for lost time and there was a lot to learn.

A necessary exposure (via music theatre) to life's remarkable complexities was finally putting a crack in my eggshell.

While touring the US with *Hairspray*, I became friends with a very special soul by the name of John Salvatore. John and I shared a connection right away. His infectiously joyous personality, mixed with an openly sardonic dark side for humor purposes, created the perfect social elixir. We became inseparable.

Which leads me to yoga.

In some circles, John is considered the golden boy teacher of hot yoga in the Western world. There are not enough superlatives to describe a class with John. He runs the gamut from professional to preposterous, all the while imparting energy and knowledge so powerful he could have an oil-rigger reciting Sanskrit while picking daisies. His popularity and influence are inarguable.

While flying on planes to different cities every week or two, I had become rundown. The remedy of choice by most cast members was to hit the bar at the start, middle, and end of each week in every new city to combat and, not surprisingly, exacerbate the original problem.

I turned to yoga.

John dragged me to class after class in city after city.

It worked. I felt lucid and invigorated.

I finished the tour, trained to become a teacher, and now own a yoga studio in Toronto, Canada.

I still act and sing, but sparingly. The rigors of owning a hot yoga business have me slipping on sweaty carpets more than walking on long red ones.

I also still practice and teach yoga regularly at the studio I own, but about a year ago, I was plagued with what I will call a "yoga virus" which led to my current (and I believe necessary) disenchantment with the word and all that surrounds it.

The only remedy for this potentially chronic yoga-hate would have to be through dissection. In the words of Robert Frost, "… the best way out is always through." The journey through would have to involve a long stare into the eyes of the dragon I once deemed a prince.

In talks with other yogis, I realized I was not the only one who was developing a peculiar hate for yoga's current identity.

The love affair had long been over.

I wanted to revive it and discerned that I could do so with a courageous exploration involving why yoga has started to suck so hard—that and musings on the influences surrounding yoga which may have helped it to start sucking so hard, all blended with perhaps the most therapeutic (in my view) approach of all: levity.

Oh, it's important to understand that there was a catalyst for my yoga-fury and *that* enabling comrade is revealed through this important disclosure: I primarily teach and practice only one form of yoga—Bikram.

Chapter 2

BIKRAM YOGA AND THE GUY WITH THE SAME NAME

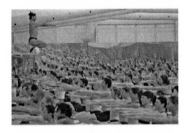

Bikram Choudhury
teaching trainees

"Corruptio optimi pessima"—*"Corruption of the best is the worst."*

—David Hume

Bikram Choudhury brought his hot yoga series from his home country of India to the United States in the 1970s. He would eventually create a series of twenty-six set postures to be practiced in a heated room for ninety minutes. He felt that these postures, performed in the same order each and every time (two sets for each), were brilliantly sequenced and the result would be a working of the entire body—inside and out—with no stone left unturned.

His instincts and expertise were dead-on.

Upon his arrival to the US, he taught the yoga for free until (the story goes) Hollywood star Shirley MacLaine, then a good friend of Bikram's, encouraged him to charge people money. It was the only way to give it credibility and enable him to expand.

Bikram and his yoga started to create a buzz, and the business of Bikram Yoga began. He started training students to be teachers of his special yoga series and that, too, took off.

At the beginning, there were only three studios teaching the Bikram method. There are now close to seven hundred around the globe with approximately half located in North America. There are also thousands of yoga teachers who only teach this method of yoga.

And there are tens of thousands of testimonials that profess, with unwavering personal clarity, how Bikram Yoga saved their lives.

I don't disagree. I will explain with distinction later on how I feel it played a large role in giving me back mine.

The Bikram Yoga series is certainly the most accessible yoga I have experienced. The postures are not easy, but they are simple. They can be slightly modified to accommodate any age, shape, or level of fitness.

The degree of difficulty, mental and physical, can be partly attributed to the fact that the room is set at 42 degrees Celsius with 40 percent humidity, easily heating up tight bodies and making the postures more accessible to those who would consider themselves inflexible.

The heat is used to increase muscle elasticity and create a cardiovascular workout. In a Bikram Yoga class, your heart can often feel like it's pounding out of your chest, and you can lose a significant amount of water weight due to the amount of sweating created; both can be tempered by the individual by not working as hard or by taking breaks.

The yoga, through its own advertised machinations, has earned a reputation for being hardass—a workout for triple-A-type personalities with a strange penchant for suffering—but most would agree that the shit works. I have read, heard, seen, and felt the evidence.

I'll save tackling the unnecessary fear factor built up around this particular yoga series for later in the book. Now that you've got an idea of the yoga, let's take a current look at the wizard behind the curtain: Bikram, the man. It's been said, "A wise man can get more use from his enemies than a fool from his friends."

I'm not about to label myself as wise, because the pressure behind fulfilling such a self-proclaimed intimation is simply more than I want to take on, but there is something about this Baltasar Gracián quote that resonates with me when I feel out my experience with Bikram, the man.

It's really not so much that Bikram is now my enemy. That would be too strong a judgment for someone from whom I have greatly benefited. But presently, I have no issue with labeling him as a huge disappointment.

Bikram, the man, has bestowed upon me—and thousands of others—the gift of a great yoga series. That will never change and, in many respects, the gifts keep on coming. But like a kid upon discovering the myth of Santa Claus, each subsequent present holds less luster with the knowledge that the mysterious and wonderful gift-giver may have morphed into a man of little moral value, to the point of being a money-grabbing narcissist.

There is also a great deal of testimony from former students accusing Bikram of being a sexual predator.

And, quite possibly, a rapist.

Nothing has been proven in court and therefore remains legally unconfirmed.

But this much can be said: The yoga Bikram brought to Western society over forty years ago remains pure. The man may not.

While Mr. Choudhury likely emanated a more evolved state of being when he brought his yoga series to the Western world, he has since been accused of falling below moral ground with the grace of an elephant onto a daisy.

I trained with Bikram during a teacher-training program that could make a college hazing look like a day at the spa.

The details of this teacher-training come later, but part of the rigorous agenda included infamous nightly lectures by the man himself, which were often just late-night ramblings on nothing more than his sexual stamina and prowess.

While the yoga remains popular and continues to hold merit due to its touted healing properties, Bikram himself seems to have become less popular.

The allure of a bad boy can lose its sheen once the word "rape" comes into the picture.

At the time of writing this, Bikram is facing sexual assault accusations from five women, some claiming they were raped.

Yup. Not funny. Not cool. Not so Namaste.

Keeping in mind that these are accusations at this point—the Los Angeles County district attorney has declined to bring any criminal charges against Bikram and all of the current cases are in civil court—it has been well-documented through numerous student/peer accounts of poor Bikram behavior that Mr. Choudhury has, perhaps, gone a little off the "deep bend" and is currently carrying a full house of hubris.

In a *Nightline* interview in 2012, Bikram defends himself against all of his detractors, explaining to the interviewer, "I never lie. I never cheat. I never hurt another spirit. I am the most spiritual man you ever met in your life. But today, you are not old, educated, smart, intelligent, wise, experienced enough to understand who I am. Maybe one of these days if you practice Bikram Yoga, you will understand that."

Here's what I understand from that statement: Nothing.

Bikram claims in the interview that half a billion people have benefited from his yoga, and in another segment, commenting on his popularity, he puts this gem out there for consideration: "People sometimes who are famous and well known, that group of people (others) get jealous. People talk bad about Jesus also."

Yes. That's true. Wars have been fought over people dissing the Lord's son. After all, he's an epic religious rock star worshipped by over a billion people worldwide; Jesus, that is. Not Bikram.

Jesus's numbers are supported by data. Bikram's? Not so much.

But how does all this happen? From my perspective, there are at least two possibilities to ponder here. One: Bikram is a victim of Western society. His original intentions were pure, profound, and purposeful, but the call of Rolls Royces and gold watches was just too alluring, and he succumbed, ultimately carving out a very dark path led by capitalism and opportunism.

Two: He's always been this person, and Western society proved to be more impressionable than he is, falling prey to Bikram's original essence, and perhaps enabling the dark seduction of some unsuspecting victims along the way.

Whichever curtain you decide to go with doesn't really matter, and there might be a few more that you could draw.

The ultimate result is unsavory.

Greatness doesn't limit itself to lovely people. There are a few biographies out there that will back this statement. Actually, most will.

The point is that even something like yoga, which usually revels in a reputation as being squeaky clean with only healing intentions can also be infiltrated and dangerously tainted by the very teachers and students that lay claim to its divinity—and all social devices to achieve this bastardization are inevitably worn out.

Human beings have a history of prioritizing their own selfish interests at the expense of the big picture. Just Google "humans and the environment."

To use Winston Churchill's assessment of Americans and broaden it to include us all, "We can always be counted on to do the right thing … once we've exhausted all other possibilities."

Yoga is not immune to the increasingly ugly imprint being left behind by human beings.

Bikram Choudhury is not the only (potentially) guilty party here, although, as of late, he's doing a great job of becoming the unchallenged poster boy. Fittingly, an article in *Yoga Journal* labeled him "Yoga's Bad Boy."

Gurus around the globe have tarnished the name of yoga by using it to transcend not adversity but common sense.

They hide behind yoga's good name and use it as a moral shield to justify indiscretions and behavior more suited to a teenage pop star than that of an enlightened master.

A man or woman of influence, charisma, and respected authority can very easily bring us under their spell using the shiny wand of trust.

When we want to trust and believe in someone, we simply will.

I did that with Bikram, but again, if I had listened to my instincts when first meeting Bikram, I would have easily surmised that something was amuck. Instead, the lure of this yoga-Medusa paralyzed my intuition, and I was loaded onto the Bikram bandwagon.

In my defense—and especially the defense of those who may have suffered or are suffering because of Bikram Choudhury—we fell in love with the yoga, not the man.

I now make a conscious and essential separation between the yoga and the man. I say all of this because I want you to do the same—regardless of what yoga you practice or decide to take up. It may be Ashtanga, Bikram, Moksha, Jivamukti, Yin, Power, Iyengar, Hot Hatha, et cetera. There are tens of styles and most are worthy of your exploration.

It doesn't matter which you choose as long as it resonates and works for *you*.

Explore the yoga on its own merits, but question everything, especially its "ambassador." I'm going to help you get the most out of a yoga practice in the second half of the book, but for now, let's continue our dive into the yoga darkness.

Note: As of September 2014, I rebranded my yoga studio and changed its name from The Bikram Yoga Centre to BeHot Yoga Toronto—a move I saw as necessary in order to accommodate evolving principles and a necessary independence that can facilitate the growth of my studio.

We still offer the Bikram style of yoga as part of our program because—to put it simply—it works.

That said, from my perspective—and the viewpoint of many of my yoga peers—the name "Bikram" has become more synonymous and representative of the healing practice that the man brought us than the man himself. It identifies the type or style of yoga being offered.

Let's not throw out the baby with the bathwater, the painting with the artist or the architecture with the architect.

If I learned powerful teachings and wisdom from a farmer who showed me how to cultivate and grow organic produce—which brought health and well-being to all who ate it—then, 40 years later, learned that the farmer was facing some very serious charges, would I separate the farm from the farmer?

Definitely.

I would continue to draw from my hard work and use the skills I had nurtured for selling that which I feel to be beneficial to people. And, just like my crops, I would grow and evolve—learning how to make everything I offer up even healthier and more accessible to the masses.

But I would leave my teacher behind.

Look, all of this is not to say that Bikram, the man, is guilty. Until proven otherwise, he is an innocent individual. That said, I am an advocate of this yoga—a yoga series that Bikram derived from the teachings of his guru, Bishnu Ghosh—because it is timeless and its powerful purity is untouchable.

If, in time, the same cannot be said for the man who pioneered it, then so be it. He must be held accountable; Bikram Choudhury that is, not the Hatha yoga series he ingeniously and unselfishly brought the western world, and which continuously transcends the potential misgivings of its troubled ambassador.

Chapter 3

ASS-ANAS AND POCKET CHANGE

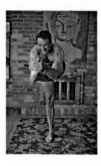

Author, Paul McQuillan, lounging around in the lobby of BeHot Yoga Toronto.

"People don't change. They just become a clearer version of who they really are."

—Unknown

There are a lot of assholes that do yoga.

I know because I've met some of them. A few practice regularly at my studio.

Unfortunately, a yoga studio is often no different than the patrons of a pub on a Saturday night. Most who frequent a pub are there for burgers, beer and a laugh, but there's always a few obnoxious drunks who make it their mission to provoke the others, contaminating the energy of the joint with their self-serving interests.

The same formula applies at a yoga studio, but it's arguably worse because some so-called "students of yoga" have a passive-aggressive side that is a little more difficult to confront and is potentially more damaging to the establishment.

Naturally, I've seen and benefited from some exemplary behavior from people at my studio. By a large percentage, they create a collective consciousness of decency that permeates the space and contributes to a healthy environment.

As wonderful as these people are, their common decency wouldn't be that interesting to write about, so let's cite a few poor examples:

Fighting over a spot in a largely unoccupied yoga room. Namaste.

Arguing with a teacher in defense of texting—during class! Namaste.

Not checking in with the front desk so as to get away with a free yoga class. Namaste.

The compassionate greeting for folks such as these? "Gone-astray."

It's important to point out that yoga doesn't have the desired effect for all who practice it and it doesn't, by its simple name, act as holy water for weirdoes. If yoga is partly defined as a diagnostic tool, bringing to the surface what may be hidden or brewing so that it may then be healed, for many it's just not working.

You don't go from jerk to Jesus with a few yoga classes. Yoga can help. For sure. But people don't change that easily and when they do, it starts small. I like to call it "pocket change."

There's an old joke: "How many therapists does it take to change a light bulb? Just one, but the bulb has to really want to change."

It's been my experience that people would like to *be* changed, but don't want to change themselves. It's simply too much work.

However, the sanctimonious will go on about how much they feel they *can* change. The problem is that if you're talking about it that much, the change is likely not that profound.

I've seen knee injuries healed, back pain obliterated, blood pressure regulated, arthritic symptoms eliminated, dramatic amounts of weight lost, and debilitating depression stabilized—all taking place with yoga being fully responsible.

But to change a person's true colors, their natural essence, their very core? That's a tall order.

Expose it? Yes. Change it? Not so much.

I have seen a lot of folks—including close friends—go through a yoga journey. The number of those yogis whose actual essence altered to the point of being poetically, significantly transformed adds up to zero.

I have become aware through my own experience that, for the most part, only traumatic events can be accredited to great change in a human being.

Many like to believe it comes from reading a great self-help book or backpacking through Europe. It really just doesn't.

These experiences can be a conduit for change but let's give true change the harrowing distinction it deserves. It's rarely a one-step process in the form of a multi-liked Facebook post.

Jeffrey A. Kottler, Ph.D, has spent 35 years interviewing people regarding their transformational experiences, and writing books about change. He writes:

> Although a small minority of people might mention something that happened in therapy, or a classroom, or formal learning experience, the vast majority of cases occurred after recovering from a challenging or even traumatic event—the death of a loved one, a major failure or disappointment, a crisis or catastrophe, a relationship or job ending, a threatening illness, or something similar.

I have a friend who was quite happy with a single life of dating in his 40s. He then had a car accident that almost took his life. He was never the same person after that accident. I witnessed him change from happy bachelor to a man on a mission for a wife and family, something that he manifested within a few years of the accident.

He changed.

One could say he moved sideways and went from happy to happy, but there was a significant change in the essence of who he was and what he wanted. You could feel how tangible it was just by being around him.

What made it all the more fascinating is that he never really spoke of it—not with any kind of pseudo-spiritual dogma, anyway. His new purpose was simple and felt.

People who have recovered from a terminal diagnosis often change.

Those who undergo intense years of psychotherapy? Sometimes.

Practicing yoga? Not really. Not by a very large percentage.

Yet, a great number of students, especially those who have just begun a yoga practice, will profess (sometimes after just one class) that they have transcended into a new world of transformation.

If you happen to be unfortunate enough to be present during one of these inauthentic happy-rants, don't take the bait. For those of you who have yet to try yoga, it might just be the final straw in confirming your decision not to; much like being on the fence about believing in Jesus, only to let your final assessment ride on the words of a man on a box in Times Square.

By all means, allow people like this to test your eye-rolling limits, but don't let them influence you with theatrical testimonials.

In the past, I've held hope that such immediate yoga enthusiasts would stretch out their change rhetoric for months to years so that actual change had a chance, but the story often plays out the same way: the bliss fades and their savior (this time yoga) loses its powers as quickly as they were deemed all-encompassing. It wasn't so much change as it was a distraction from the pain. This isn't necessarily a bad thing. It's just not consistent and it sure isn't deep.

Often, if not always, the best thing we can do for ourselves if we partake in a regular yoga practice is to get in the room and shut up.

The benefits of such a simple action are potentially profound. Your attitude might change. Your awareness. Your perspective. Your choices. Naturally, your body will also benefit.

But you will still be you.

Yoga can lead you to understanding your essence. You may even come to the conclusion that you're a bit of an asshole. But at least then you can make a conscious choice not to be, with yoga being instrumental in bringing that awareness to light and that shift possible.

Call me crazy, but I see all of this as good news. Yoga can do something as simple and extraordinary as clearing the view.

Don't let the pretentious promise of change through yoga cloud the mirror of daily possibility with expectation and unneeded pressure.

Embrace the little things. They add up. Maybe even to change.

Chapter 4

THE UNTAUGHT TEACHER

"I have noticed that teachers get exciting confused with boring a lot."

—Sara Pennypacker, *The Talented Clementine*

I didn't start teaching yoga until about a year ago.

This is an unfortunate admission given the fact that I've been teaching officially since 2006, the same year I graduated from Bikram Yoga Teacher Training.

I spoke a lot of words to many rooms full of people for years, but I never taught.

In retrospect, not only did I not know what I was doing, I actually could have been causing people harm.

And I'm not alone.

If you happen to be one of my students during that time, I'm sorry if this disclosure sends chills down your potentially misaligned spine.

The further truth is that while I'm embarrassed that I called myself a teacher when I came out of training, it's highly unlikely that I caused anyone injury because I didn't physically make posture adjustments to my students in the first few years.

The teacher-training program at Bikram Yoga (which is by no means the only program guilty of the following) is a yoga factory which exists to maximize the number of Bikram teachers in the world as quickly as possible—getting impressionable yoga-baked souls to feel as though they are actually yoga teachers—so that they can then spread the yoga love to the masses with the grace and finesse of a drunken teenager.

This is done with a memorized, assigned Bikram "dialogue" (actually a monologue because there is no verbal interaction, only recitation) which is one or two pages long for each of the 26 postures and two breathing exercises offered up in the series.

When you graduate, you stand in front of a classroom of people in your studio of choice and you say the "dialogue."

You're a yoga teacher.

The bodies move and people do what you say, even if the grammar for some of the dialogue is purposefully wrong, broken and somewhat misleading; even if you don't really see the bodies because you're so in your head; even if you are simply a programmed machine that has been exported (immediately following graduation) from the training location to Australia, Canada, Japan, Great Britain—or tens of other countries—to string words together and speak a whole lot o' wrong.

The true crime here is that it actually works. People buy it.

The Bikram "dialogue" is laced with gems like, "grab your elbows each other", "pull more harder" and compassionate ditties such as "your back is going to hurt like hell."

It's a testament to the yoga that students actually adhere to the disjointed instruction. Not the words.

And usually not the teacher.

Not the new ones, anyway. It could be argued that you gotta start somewhere, but when you're pretending to be the medium for a student's healing through yoga and orchestrating the potential for major re-construction in a person's physiology, I'm gonna go ahead and say that memorization should not be the primary tool of choice, particularly when it instructs you that "your back is going to hurt like hell."

When doing a yoga posture, nothing should hurt like hell. Nothing.

So there it be. The template for teacher success: Memorization and dictation.

As an actor, if I didn't put substance, meaning and understanding behind the words I memorized, I usually either didn't get the job, or I simply sucked at the job I was doing.

At my yoga training, we learned very little about the actual postures we were going to dictate. There was no time—another alarming fact given that we were in the yoga training facility for upwards of 12-15 hours a day for nine solid weeks.

We did two 90-minute classes a day, some basic anatomy study which made no link to the yoga and four to six hours of "posture clinics", which is a deceiving term because it actually involves sitting and listening to other would-be teachers reciting a different verbal instruction for a posture each day by rote.

Thus, the bulk of your time was spent listening to others say what they memorized.

This was not the stuff yoga dreams were made of. Time consuming, yes. Productive and inspiring? I've felt more sense of accomplishment from watching episodes of Seinfeld—a show about nothing.

The dialogue was mostly written and approved by Bikram himself and as blatantly incorrect as much of it is, he stands by it with the same conviction as his innocence on rape allegations.

I hope that he is just guilty of spreading bad grammar around the world (a large enough crime in my books), but alas, bad words often lead to bad actions.

If there is a better example of "commercializing" yoga for the sake of profit (tuition for each wannabe teacher at the time of writing is $11,400 USD with two/room accommodation), I have yet to find one, but again, my teacher-training experience is limited to just Bikram yoga.

While the Bikram training may be comparatively more physically and mentally arduous than many programs, which require your time on a few weekends to pronounce you a teacher, that doesn't mean it's the most credible.

Of all the teachers of different yoga factions I talked to for the purposes of this book, not one convinced me that they had undergone a training program extensive or thorough enough to prove themselves worthy of being qualified to actually teach the complexities of this ancient art form.

The unwarranted proliferation of largely incompetent yoga teachers is such a crime it should be considered malpractice.

Some teachers from the wild yoga world of the west are actually very good. They are good because they work diligently and with purpose to become believably good at what they do; and it is my argument that they likely already had an innate sense of the body, movement and (as is the partial theme) instincts that are conducive to becoming a teacher of yoga.

In short, it may be their calling.

I believe that we're all born for a purpose and that your calling could be largely obvious. Good with numbers? Perhaps being an accountant is a piece of your puzzle. Born with a great singing voice? Could be a clue to attend the local "Idol" auditions.

But I know this: You're not a yoga teacher just because you say you are.

That's a declaration that could hurt a lot of people.

Now, a distinction is necessary. I'm not arguing that yoga doesn't work. It does, when taught correctly. But some of the teaching methods are about as ill advised as allowing a lousy mid-wife to deliver the next King of Siam.

The yoga is the King of Siam. The teaching methods are the lousy midwife. Just clarifying.

I am a teacher now. Not a great one. But I am helping people and I'm doing so through a knowledge of the postures which I formulated through the years after I graduated; but when I think back just a few years ago to the dude who taught with a bunch of words, no heart, no experience, cocky swagger and no presence, I'm embodied by the kind of shame that would make Richard Nixon feel like Mother Teresa.

I've since forgiven myself. I really would like to believe that I am now helping people through an ever-growing mix of experience and humility. I don't know everything and I certainly don't pretend to be the back alley Buddha that people seek out at times, but much like my post-college days, it's only through actual experience and the exchange of arrogance for intuition that I have arrived at a place where I can call myself a taught teacher.

You can benefit greatly from yoga and from an experienced yoga teacher. It may be like finding an honest politician, but they're out there. Just do your best to identify and abandon anyone who pretends to have all the yoga answers. Run fast and far…into the arms of another teacher and, if necessary, rinse and repeat.

All professions ride the same sliding scale of credibility. Yoga teachers are no different.

Chapter 5

GURU BE GONE

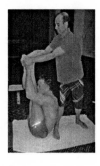

Paul, training
with respected
Hatha yoga expert,
Tony Sanchez,
in Mexico, 2014.

"When Chuck Norris does yoga, there is only one guru:
Chuck Norris."

—Chuck Norris joke. One of thousands.

I n this information age, it is becoming clearer that individuals
are more autonomous than ever, and we are actually entering
into an era where mentors are becoming less common.
The same applies in the yoga world. As yogis develop a better
understanding of whatever yoga they are practicing and begin
to comprehend the basic form of postures and the will required
to execute them, so-called gurus will become somewhat scarce.

I've always been of the opinion that admiring someone too much can have an adverse effect on the admirer because it relieves him or her of the accountability accompanied by potential greatness.

Greatness can be a daunting responsibility, no doubt. It would seem much easier to let others be giants and simply follow in their path, all the while staying just below the bar they have set.

Too many budding protégés have fallen prey to this common formula, but I really believe the tide is changing.

As an example, I have yogis asking me well-educated questions regarding Hatha yoga, and when I give what I believe to be a definitive response, it is followed by yet another astute question, taking us further into the subject. My word is not taken as fact and if there's even a suspicion of anything dubious being offered in my teachings, a quick Google search that evening will bring the student back—questioning my possibly outdated and suspect knowledge—the very next day.

Discernment is a greater part of the learning process now. It's a positive and valuable evolvement.

When I trained with Tony Sanchez in Mexico in the early part of 2014, his humility, openness and accessibility were refreshing. His teaching styles were the antithesis of Bikram's who clearly favors a more dictatorial approach. Tony was the Switzerland to Bikram's Nazi Germany.

As a matter of fact, some of Tony's first words were, "I want you to question *everything*." And we did. We came at him with years of brewing scrutiny surrounding everything we thought we knew—and he calmly disarmed us with the most powerful weapons in his personal arsenal: knowledge, mutual respect, experience and kindness.

It's possible that mentoring will not die if the way we mentor can evolve and become less about superiority and more about the depth of experience matched with facts and a comprehensive understanding of the subject. Add mutual respect to the mix and the makings of a meaningful relationship between teacher and student will simply eliminate the unnecessary and somewhat pressure-laden title of mentor.

In the subject of yoga, the guru-eclipse will help more people move towards practicing for the first time because they may just be less intimidated by the self-righteous salad-eater they envision to be their yoga teacher.

I have many friends who won't go near a yoga studio because the pretentiousness they experienced during their first few visits was enough to make them want to kick the teacher in the face, leaving a considerably ugly carbon footprint.

Understandable. Just recently, while vacationing in another city, my girlfriend and I listened to a yoga teacher go on annoyingly about how important it was to her that the studio go paperless, not realizing that we just watched her pull into her parking spot in a gas-guzzling truck so big it could only be used to carry the staggering weight of her hypocrisy.

I know that hundreds of Bikram's loyal followers are now dumbfounded—to the point of being completely heartbroken—by the mere notion that the man behind the yoga they love may not be the respected, lead-by-example guru he once was. The flies around him are too many to ignore.

But if there's a silver lining here, it's that they now have to move forward with a platform constructed of their own principles. They have been pushed into a corner in which a bright light is shining down upon them and questions that can no longer be delegated to the Bikram camp are being pointedly asked.

This presents a wonderful opportunity for ownership and hopefully a clearer understanding of how to become the shepherd and not just another one of the sheep.

Whether voluntarily stepping away from the reliance of mentorship or being forcibly pushed beyond it, the result can be delightfully liberating.

You're the guru now.

With any bloody war, there are often a few unsuspecting casualties. So, as we continue to drive a stake into the heart of yoga's society-born bastard child, it seems only fitting to watch calmly as the sun rises in the background and burns out the eyes of its brethren, the bogus guru.

Chapter 6

PAGING DOCTOR DOES-LITTLE

"Though the doctors treated him and gave him medications to drink, he nevertheless recovered."

—Leo Tolstoy, War and Peace

am not a doctor. But sometimes I play one in real life.

I'm also not a disciple or spiritual conduit for the teachings of Jesus, Buddha, Mohammed, Ghandi or Moses.

But the leap from yoga teacher to medical expert or great guru of wisdom is not as large as one might believe.

With the simple credential of understanding a few postures, a yoga teacher can suddenly rise to that of sage-like status and carry brain-surgeon bravado.

You see, the problem is that western culture's yoga students place a lot of faith in their teacher, arguably more than they should. After only a few classes, they are often putting the finishing touches on a vessel of trust with broad swipes of glossy credibility. They then board the yoga ship without question and it sails into the clear waters of possibility.

The problem is that they may have just boarded the Titanic.

To be a doctor, you need years of intense study and practice. To be an iconic figure of enlightenment, you usually need to go through an epic journey that ends with your crucifixion, assassination or simple exhaustion from wandering through a desert for 40 years.

But to be a yoga-doctor/guru, you just have to read a few self-help books and know that ice is good for swelling.

Here's a typical student/teacher exchange:

Student: "I seem to have injured my back."

Teacher: "Does it hurt when you do backbends?"

Student: "No."

Teacher: "Forward bends?"

Student: "Yes."

Teacher: "Okay, when you're going into your forward bends and it starts to hurt, pull back."

Student: "Okay. Is there anything I should do for it?"

Teacher: "When you get home, ice it."

Student: "Anything else?"

Teacher: "Well, back pain often manifests through a fear of not being supported by the universe and repressed rage. Know that the world and the people around you love you. Oh, and ya might want to take a look at forgiving your mother. That's likely the root cause, unless of course you've yet to deal with your paralyzing fear of rejection and abandonment. (Pause) Any questions?"

Okay, I made the last part up, but my point is likely made.

When you start yoga, or if you're already benefiting from a yoga practice, it's important to understand that your yoga teacher is not Hugh Laurie on *House*.

One of the wisest bits of advice I have ever received was also the most simple: "Get people to do what they do," followed by, "show me what a man does most and I'll show you what he does best."

In legal trouble? Get a good lawyer. Muscles tight? A good RMT.

But it's wise not to fall prey to thinking that a yoga teacher can help you understand why there's blood in your urine.

See. A. Doctor.

Take your pick: Naturopath, GP, acupuncturist. Some are very good and—just like yoga teachers—some will kinda suck.

Nonetheless, the dangerous notion that yoga can take the place of the great advancements in modern medicine and the doctors who diligently practice it only has a spot in one place: The morgue.

We will explore the healthy mix of yoga and doctors who prescribe it later as well as the reality of lousy doctors and the pills they irresponsibly and copiously prescribe; but for now, understanding the difference between a doctor and a yoga teacher is as important as the simple understanding that just because George Bush was president of the most powerful country in the world doesn't mean he wasn't a complete idiot.

Chapter 7

GOOD GOD, YOGA

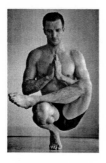

Paul in
toe-stand.

*"I'm not normally a praying man, but if you're up there,
please save me Superman!"*

—Homer Simpson

I n a chapter of his book, *God Is Not Great*, the late
Christopher Hitchens—known for his intellectualism
and religious irreverence—answers a hypothetical
question: If he were alone in an unfamiliar city at night and
a group of strangers began to approach him, would he feel
safer or less safe knowing that these men had just come from
a prayer meeting?

Hitchens answers, "Just to stay within the letter 'B', I have actually had that experience in Belfast, Beirut, Bombay, Belgrade, Bethlehem and Baghdad. In each case, I would feel immediately threatened if I thought that the group of men approaching me in the dusk were coming from a religious observance."

He gives detailed descriptions of the varied social and political tensions within these cities, which he personally attributes to religion. He has thus "not found it a prudent rule to seek help as the prayer meeting breaks up."

It's a sobering point.

It's also best not to seek out the help of religion when it comes to a yoga practice.

Yoga and religion don't mix. Except they do.

Some zealots will do their best to link their religious beliefs with their yoga practice—and then yours.

Don't drink the Kool-Aid.

Yoga is about freeing the body and mind, not institutionalizing them. I fear that religion is just too formal a construct to compliment a yoga practice. Yoga is conducive to creating universal acceptance of all who live on this earth, not just a select million or two based on specified (sometimes dictated) beliefs.

I am not taking a stance against religion, let's be clear. There are many who use their religion of choice as a personal beacon to guide them through life, and when they do so without the need to enlist others—all the while maintaining their individual integrity and honoring the religion that resonates for them—I have no doubt that it can be a useful tool for faith.

Many benefit from their religious choices, but some will argue that yoga takes its roots from religious principles and doctrines.

It doesn't.

There are many assertions regarding the origin of yoga, but despite a self-serving attempt in recent years by The American Hindu Foundation to lay its claim on yoga and give it a religious moniker, attaching religion to yoga has been seen as a futile endeavor.

Besides, even if a sensible jury found yoga guilty of mixing carelessly with religion, the decision can be overturned. By you.

It will not behoove you physically, mentally or spiritually to mix religion with yoga. Red bull and vodka is a safer mix. It's like putting Mozart and Kenny G. in the same room. It's just not advisable, necessary or productive. Only dissonance will ensue.

Yoga is a spiritual practice, not a religious one.

I was raised Catholic, dragged to church most Sundays, and even endured a few strange but undamaging years as an altar boy (an accomplishment given the history of abuse in that environment) until the liberating feeling of subjective thought freed itself cautiously within me like a prisoner from an unlocked jail cell.

Around the year of my 16th birthday, I began silently questioning what I felt to be the highly illogical and archaic principles of the Catholic Church.

I may have been positively influenced by a stepmother who—after serving the church as a nun for 20 years—made the courageous decision to leave, but nonetheless remains a devout Catholic to this day.

She came into my life when I was around 12 and explained later that the whole scene just became too political and self-serving for her liking. She felt that serving God as a layperson was more her style. Good thing too because she met my father just a few years after kicking her habit and they married not long after that.

I say without a hint of irony that she is a saint of a woman, and if I actually did believe in heaven, the serendipitous and timely matchup of her and my father would have been what sealed the deal.

But I don't.

I sure wish I did. Sitting in a pew for an hour a week and eating a few wafers of unsalted bread doesn't seem quite as arduous as following my belief of backbends as a portal to the human spirit.

I suppose both paths carry their weight, but sharing that weight would be even more daunting.

One could get very intimidated and confused by the ill-advised hybrid of religion and yoga, so keep them separate. If you can, you must. It will actually benefit your yoga practice to do so and, if you do adhere to a certain religion, it will only create more clarity with regards to your beliefs once you leave the yoga room.

Believe what you believe, but in order to start or maintain a lucid, beneficial yoga practice, the complexities and inherent controversies surrounding religion could easily handicap the healing potentialities of a non-denominational yoga practice.

The unfortunate reality is this: On the best of days, religion remains partially synonymous with war, violence, hate and intolerance in the world. It's not the tainted backdrop we want to look at it when we practice yoga in front of a mirror.

Therefore, as part of our yoga exorcism—and our quest to expel all impurities from the word and infuse it with a raw simplicity—it's important to ask religion if it will politely leave the room.

If you're a religious person, there's no need to feel offended. If you are, let's hope we don't run into each other on the street at the end of one of your prayer meetings.

Here is my prayer: That you understand that I am not attacking your religion, but merely suggesting that yoga and religion remain uncompromisingly autonomous; a distinction that will only serve you, your yoga practice and perhaps even your religion.

Chapter 8

SMOKE AND MIRRORS

"The opposite of courage is not cowardice, it is conformity.
Even a dead fish can go with the flow."
—Jim Hightower

M ore people are doing yoga now in America than ever before.

Yoga Journal released a "Yoga in America" study in 2012 which shows that 20.4 million Americans practice yoga compared to 15.8 million from the previous 2008 study, an increase of 29 percent. In addition, practitioners spend $10.3 billion USD a year on yoga classes and products. The previous estimate from the 2008 study was $5.7 billion USD.

This could be construed as a good thing, of course.

But just because something grows in popularity, does not mean it's wise to put a blanket of benefit over the entire activity.

Cigarette smoking also reached its peak in popularity in the 60s, the same decade that a man first landed on the moon. Sometimes, stupid is as smart does.

"Stupid is" refers to smoking. "Smart does" is the moon-landing feat. Just clarifying.

I have already begun to take the clear stance that yoga is beneficial to one's health, and I will enhance that position further after we deconstruct all the hype and confusion, but the point I wish to spark up is that it's not wise to do it just because everyone else does.

Smoking cigarettes is a stupid choice, often taken up by smart people who succumb to following the fold.

Yoga is a smart choice, often abandoned or never begun because it requires qualities that smoking does not: work ethic, dedication and, of course, a desire to practice yoga.

Some people simply don't have the aspiration, curiosity and commitment to make it a regular discipline in their lives—and the very thought of a yoga practice fills them with gross disdain. In this case, they're never going to benefit from yoga based on this simple conclusion: They don't want to.

Now, that may sound like a lot of smoke and mirrors and you may be wondering if I got high before writing this—and while you'll never really know the answer to that question, let's use "weed" and its rampant use as an excuse to blow more smoke.

Marijuana is proven to help individuals suffering from the chronic pain that comes with disease; however, for many healthy people, it simply serves as a great way to feel pleasure and, perhaps, act as an enabler of the right-to-*not*-work movement.

Yup. Some people just do it because it makes them feel good. If it didn't, they wouldn't smoke it. As Barack Obama once cheekily pointed out in a news interview, "I inhaled… frequently. That was the point."

Which brings me to my point. Yoga can also help with disease and pain—without other unpleasant side effects—but the process may not be as enjoyable or as simple as a few inhales. It takes work. In this case, it is a means to an end.

Yoga is practiced to make you feel good.

The Bikram yoga series was originally designed to heal injuries. That's why the postures are quite simple and accessible. But if you're in perfect health and don't suffer from pain or injuries, why are you doing it? The obvious answer would be for maintenance and prevention, but if the practice of yoga itself is something you just do because you feel you have to, it may not be serving its purpose.

There is value in wanting to.

Yoga should be practiced with the ultimate goal of making you feel good and part of that equation is embracing the process.

I'll be the first to say that my yoga training was stupidly excessive. From my experience, there is NO benefit to 3 hours of hot yoga a day for 9 weeks. Such extremes only further the common sense principle that anything to excess is probably not a good idea, and may just do more harm than good.

I was dehydrated, stiff, grumpy, bloated and embarrassingly gassy for the entire duration.

A *means* to an end? That was the pill being shoved down our throats.

I saw it as more of a *pain* in the end, the equivalent of having a needle jabbed into a different part of my body until there were no veins left, at which point, they just kept jabbing anyway.

Dramatic? Maybe. It's possible that 30 years in theatre leaves me (and you) prone to some harmless embellishment, but for those of you who have been through a Bikram yoga training, it may not be seen as much of an exaggeration.

To further my point, I personally know many teachers who graduated from that training only to never teach or practice yoga again.

They hate it.

I've also seen many others give yoga an honest effort and come to the salient, coherent conclusion that it is just not for them.

Because *they* hate it.

I agree with the philosophy that many of our decisions and actions in this life contain either the energy of faith or fear. If the fear of doing yoga cannot be overcome or—if after giving it a good go—it only instills more anxiety, fear, expectation or mental anguish (for whatever reason), it's clear: Yoga is not for you.

You may not need to go through the cathartic process of killing yoga and then taking part in its resurrection because, for you, it never left the womb.

A life without yoga can still be a good one.

No, seriously, I'm not high. It can.

Chapter 9

#YOGA—A FEAR OF "LIKES"

"Distracted from distraction by distraction."
—T.S. Eliot

witter and Facebook can saturate and destroy a healthy subject like Coca-Cola on bran flakes.

To use either of these popular platforms to help establish your understanding of yoga would be like using a hammer to open a fine bottle of Chardonnay.

For those that are impressionable enough to go on the ride, social media—in its current sultry state of provocation—can take a vulnerable and authentic art form like yoga and turn it into an overnight fad that, according to a recent study by an unknown Facebook friend, (with wall-to-wall research collected from hours of newsfeeds) actually causes premature death and, perhaps more gravely, persistent self-righteousness.

And it has to be true. It got "liked" and "shared" by that guy's friend who used to be a yoga teacher but died one night of chronic Savasana.

This entire journey ends with a few hundred "likes" and a cyber-burning of virtual yoga mats.

And just like that, yoga is dead.

But it kind of had it coming. Yoga studios are businesses after all and with each greasing of the post-pole, they slide further down into a world that confuses flirtation with unprotected penetration.

Conversely, with social media acting as its shady ambassador, yoga—any type, depending on the day—can be lifted to heights of credibility that impose a sense of deification upon it that does not serve the purpose of making it largely accessible to the masses.

Much like yoga and religion, social media and yoga don't know how to play nice. Somebody needs to leave the sandbox.

Here's my confession: I utilize social media all the time to promote my business. I use sexy yoga pictures, motivational mantras, stories of transformation, testimonials from celebrity yogis and—ironically, but very effectively—comedic quotes or cartoons that take the piss out of yoga.

I play the game because in our consumer culture it's a game that simply must be played. It's a silly means to a productive end. Credibility be damned!

When we immunize, a poison is often used as a part of the potion. The poison plays a part in protecting us from the sickness. That said, our awareness of the ingredients of a flu shot could help us responsibly determine whether or not to get one. Depending upon your view, it may hurt or it may help.

Facebook, Twitter, Instagram, Linkedin and the twelve other cyber-media outlets which may have made their debut in the past ten minutes can be used to provide us with connection, information and harmless folly—but don't forget that there's a bit of poison in every poke.

The biggest problem with social media is that posts, tweets and responses to both do not have to be accompanied by the accountability that actual presence and human interaction demand.

There's a personal and compassionate touch that is lost somewhere between the heart and the computer screen, tablet or smart phone as people freely and often callously spin their (world wide) web. We all know of good people being tormented or uncharacteristically becoming the tormentor as a result of doling out advice or commentary through social media while hiding behind their protective cyber-wall.

Ironically, social media can be tagged as the least evolved form of communication because the effort behind it is weak and the connection impersonal.

I would like everyone who ever posts or tweets something cheeky, controversial or downright mean to ask themselves if they would have the courage to stand in front of a room of people and dictate the same words they so effortlessly put forth through a social media platform; and if the answer is "yes", they have to tell me "yes" to my face and then I get to set up the meeting, choosing other guilty perpetrators to pack the gallery. The room would likely be filled with cowardice silence. And yes, I would be there as well—given *my* past improprieties.

Learning about yoga—or even looking for validation of the type of yoga you practice— through social media may be the equivalent of learning how to dance the tango by reading a book on how to dance the mambo; there's going to be more than a few missteps, confusion will ensue, then suddenly something that could have been personally healing and held close with deference is tainted with the carelessness of public un-appeal.

The validation comes from you and your physical experience, not through callous commentary from strangers or the estranged.

Bullying in our modern day has actually increased dramatically since the introduction and proliferation of social media.

To cite just one of many examples, according to a study entitled, "Teens, Kindness and Cruelty on Social Network Sites" by the Pew Research Center's Internet & American Life Project, which surveyed 800 children between the ages of 12 and 17, a large percentage of teens admit they have seen cruelty online; of those who witnessed it, 21 percent said they joined in the harassment.

Three out of 10 girls ages 12 to 13 said they have experienced mostly unkind treatment on social networks— the most negative response of any group of youth, according to the report.

It would come as no surprise that adults are not immune to this cruelty; nor is any subject matter, including yoga.

Everything and everyone is a potential target on social media.

If you practice yoga or decide to start, keep the path pure by brushing aside the cynicism synonymous with social media.

It could easily get you bent out of shape.

Chapter 10

BOURBON AND BACKBENDS

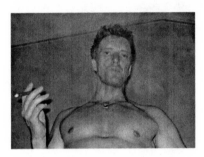

Vacationing (and cigar-smoking) in
La Romana, Dominican Republic.

*"Every form of addiction is bad, no matter whether the
narcotic be alcohol or morphine or idealists."*
—Carl Jung

There *is* such a thing as too much yoga. Anything given
an extreme amount of governance over our bodies can
begin to take an unhealthy stronghold that does not
adhere to balance and moderation.

Being moderate has been a lifelong struggle for me.

My dear late father was an alcoholic while I grew up
and I'm more than a little aware of the reality that I am

predisposed to being vulnerable to the seductive dance of addiction.

I do my very best to temper that exposure with moderation, not only in drinking alcohol, but in everything I do, and that includes yoga. Most of the time it works, but sometimes, well…

It. Just. Doesn't.

I get drunk. I eat too much chocolate. I drink too much coffee. I smoke pot. I take a sleeping pill. I smoke a cigar. I project an angry mood onto the students I'm teaching. I get inconsolably depressed. I shut out my friends and emotionally distance myself from my family and my partner.

And yes, sometimes, I do too much yoga.

Balance will always be my north star, but occasionally my moral compass fails me. When it does, getting back on track usually has something to do with self-forgiveness and setting a new template that may help guide me a little better this time 'round.

In the Hollywood movie *Unfaithful* (2002), the female character—a married woman played by Diane Lane—is wooed by a younger man and begins a love affair that ends tragically.

I remember listening to interviews following the film in which the director explains that he wanted to be sure in his narrative that there was no distinct, obvious motive for the affair; a happily married woman—in love with her husband—simply allows her desires to be satiated by a man she finds strongly compelling.

In Diane Lane's interview, she was asked why or how this could happen (for her character) in what appeared to be an emotionally healthy climate of dedication and contentment with her husband. Her answer was simple:

"Sometimes we fail in our convictions."

Hey, guess what? Sometimes, we fail in our convictions.

So be it. But when we think we've found a solution for extreme or addictive behavior by exchanging it for another form of damaging conduct, we're moving chairs around on the Titanic.

We all know the stories. An alcoholic trades his booze addiction for two packs of cigarettes a day and 12 cups of coffee, mistaking the move sideways as a revelatory progression.

It's important to see yoga as a middle path. Give it too much weight and you risk burnout from the very activity you turn to for energy and focus. It is one of the many tools used to carve out a good life—along with diet, other forms of exercise, and healthy relationships—but it's about as much of a cure-all as that Sunday morning Bloody Mary.

Like anything else, yoga can become a disturbing and damaging form of addiction that can breed obsessive behavior and extremism.

This is illustrated no better than in the insightful book *Hell-Bent* by Benjamin Lorr, in which the author goes through excessive amounts of (Bikram) yoga training and furthers his obsession with yoga workshops that promise euphoria through unnecessary—and potentially harmful—amounts of backbends.

But Mr. Lorr, in his noble and courageous quest for yoga-truth, also presents a balanced point of view from others. He quotes Dennis Dronjic who—after getting into a motorcycle accident so grave that doctors said he would never walk again—exclaims with reasonable perspective:

> The yoga didn't save my life. That was the emergency response team, the surgeons, the rehab specialists. The yoga didn't give me the drive to recover. That came from some place inside me. What the yoga did is allow me to use the life I had been given back. And what's the point otherwise? What good is having a body if you can't use it?

Extremes of any kind can produce unwanted results.

Too often, I can only observe cautiously as I watch yet another new student place all their eggs in the yoga basket. It misses the point because—instead of instilling faith in themselves—they are making yoga responsible for their happiness.

Nothing can carry that much weight alone. The bottom usually falls out and the inevitable conclusion is that perhaps yoga's not all it's cracked up to be.

It is. But much like you, it doesn't like that kind of pressure. When yoga is practiced relentlessly without paying attention to the very body you are working to keep healthy, the results can be damaging.

As a studio owner, I witness students who are obviously doing too much yoga for all the wrong reasons, namely to support other dysfunctions—image issues and eating disorders to list just a few.

Yes, even yoga can be an enabler.

The higher ground of connection, balance, awareness and health is rarely enjoyed in yoga when the fog of excess rolls in and blinds us from a clear path of moderation.

The NCADD (National Council on Alcoholism and Drug Dependence) lists yoga as being helpful in the recovery of addiction:

> Yoga cultivates bodily awareness in a kind, nurturing way. It allows students to start connecting with the body and breath and learn to sit and look within. Compassion for oneself arises and with it, a new ability to deal with stressful situations, leading to positive change.

They don't say how *much* yoga (see Pattie Lovett-Reid's cautionary tale in the foreword of this book). And what about yoga for yoga addiction? I can't seem to find a study on that.

Oh, and guess what The NCADD *doesn't* list yoga as? A cure.

If you want to get obsessed with something, start with moderation. It will take the expectation and pressure off you and yoga.

Then, if you occasionally do too much yoga and have to pull yourself back, or you don't do enough and miss a few classes here and there, well…

Sometimes people fail in their convictions.

Movie spoiler alert! By the way, Richard Gere (who plays Diane Lane's husband in *Unfaithful*) failed in his convictions as well, but it could be argued that he went a bit too far and entered into a place of extremes. Upon learning of the affair and confronting his wife's lover, he builds into a fit of rage and kills him with a snow globe.

Ouch. Being Canadian, that scene hit me hard. We *love* our snow globes.

Doing too much yoga rarely leads to murder—again, I couldn't find any studies—but if not done responsibly and in moderation, it could end up killing the very balance you're trying to achieve for a healthy life.

Chapter 11

NO COMPETITION

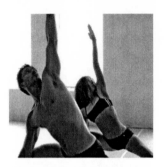

Paul with Teshia Maher, yoga
teacher and 2012 Eastern
Canada Asana Champion.

com·pe·ti·tion /kämpə'tiSHən/noun: The activity or condition of striving to gain or win something by defeating or establishing superiority over others.
—Oxford Dictionary

There's a third guilty party in the "I don't mix with yoga" formula, and while it would seem like an open and shut case of obvious conviction for the accused, strangely, the trial lingers on while the jury remains largely baffled and mixed in judgment.

The perpetrator has a name: Competition. But it's only when paired with its unsuspecting partner that the crime is given its weighty cross:

Yoga Competition.

An oxymoron to many, a celebration to others, but a reality nonetheless.

The United States Yoga Federation (USA Yoga) has run regional and national championships for 11 years. "Winners" are sent to compete at the global level.

In 2014, London, England hosted the World Yoga Sports Championship run by the International Yoga Sports Federation. The ultimate goal of all of this is to eventually get yoga recognized as an Olympic sport.

Full disclosure: In Toronto, which I have made home for close to 30 years, I was the Master of Ceremonies for a few of the Canadian Eastern Regional Yoga Asana Championships.

I admit this because I don't want it to seem hypocritical when I present my argument against such events. I can only say that, even back then, an underlying hesitance was lying dormant within me regarding yoga competitions.

Those initial feelings of quiet disagreement have since come to fruition and blossomed into full contempt.

The feelings are the equivalent of being a professional basketball player in the middle of a championship game, only to come to the sobering and somewhat untimely epiphany that you actually hate basketball.

In 2014, I chose to not support the local competition with sponsorship through my studio as I had done reluctantly in the past. A few other studio owners—upset with this decision and incorrectly seeing it as a personal shunning of their beliefs—did their passive-aggressive best to ostracize me and label me an uncooperative troublemaker with a selfish agenda.

My only agenda was to listen to my instincts, which finally told me with unwavering clarity, that a yoga competition might just discredit the original purpose of yoga, placing it in an arena of lions and warriors—a setting that would not seem conducive to the feeling of personal growth potentially obtained through yoga in a safe environment.

Bettering one's self through yoga is a subjective journey in which the devices wielded need not consist of sharp edges. It would seem more productive to don the tools of acceptance and compassion than that of comparison, which can enhance—or at least subconsciously encourage—self-judgment.

As for yoga as an Olympic sport, how will the judges accurately assess the degree and depth of meditation that is being reached in each posture, given that transcending thought is a key ingredient to growth in an asana?

Sure, the posture may be "performed"—another troublesome word in this context—with magnificent feats of flexibility and strength and perfect form, but how do we know the competitor has completely arrived at a sense of detachment—the measurement of which, I assume, would be quite difficult.

If yoga does become an Olympic sport, I would anticipate it carrying with it as much or more controversy as that of ice dancing. Even if the judges have reached a personal level of transcendence in themselves and starred in multiple sequels of *The Matrix*, it may be a little more than tricky to recognize and score each yogi based on their subjective level of enlightenment—yet another comparison that would be the equivalent of corn and oranges. Both good. But which is *better*?

And when the yoga champions are somehow determined, are they crowned with the spiritual distinction and loftiness of the Pope, Mother Theresa or the second coming of Jesus? After all, having a winner would denote a sense of arrival and completion as opposed to the ongoing and endless journey that is an integral part of a personal yoga practice.

Then again, maybe the end of the world's troubles is not through us acting responsibly as individuals and creating our own personal paths of awareness. Maybe we need to put all the pressure on someone else who is clearly just *better* at it than we are.

Phew. That's a relief.

I just changed my mind. I LOVE yoga competitions! Bring me my Queen.

Chapter 12

_**MY**_ YOGA!

"You have to do your own growing, no matter how tall
your grandfather was."
                    —Abraham Lincoln

Sometimes, for the sake of levity, I get excited while teaching a strong class of yogis and exclaim proudly: "Yeah, that's right. Make that yoga your bitch."

My intention is never actually to encourage even the possibility that yoga can be owned or possessed with the same peculiar dedication as that of an adult to a stuffed toy.

Much like the toy, whose furry umbilical cord needs to be severed by its owner before the late teen years, a separation from yoga is necessary in order to establish a perspective that promotes growth. (By the way, if you're one of those obsessed-by-their-stuffed-pet people, I apologize.)

And now—after a suitably long pause—I retract that apology. It's strange behavior. Please cut it out.

Entitlement to yoga is a dangerous path littered with sanctimonious affirmations and uninspiring, clichéd mantras. It's no basis for an authentic connection and it's a relationship that will end poorly.

For you.

Yoga will be fine. It recognizes when it's in the deep end of your emotionally-polluted waters and it swims away safely, all the while watching you drown in your self-made sea of asana.

It's a sad, but predictable tale.

You'll feel hurt by yoga in the end. It will be hard for you to stay friends. Somewhere between sweating on your rubber and spraying it down, you smothered yoga.

You just wanted too much, too fast. You got too close.

It's sad because you thought yoga was the one. But yoga was unfaithful. Extremely so. It selfishly served its own needs and couldn't commit to just you.

It maintained its endless patterns of deep breathing with others and not feeling guilty afterward.

How could it have ended like this, you mull bitterly. You were always there for yoga. Seven days a week. Sometimes you did it twice a day. Was yoga faking it? It seemed mutual. Sincere.

Things were going so well.

Then came yoga's need for a cross-legged-sit-down relationship talk and—like a barrage of yoga blocks to the head and straps to the heart—out came this admission:

"I need more space," yoga said. "Some time to breathe."

"What?" you protest. "When did this happen?"

Yoga explains that you've changed. It still loves you but it's not *in* love with you. It suggests you both start seeing other people. It needs to branch out and use its eight special limbs to entangle with others.

You're pissed. You turn to your friends to enroll them in yoga's misgivings and betrayal.

Sadly, this relationship and all its Prana-drama have already tired them out.

They've listened to your stories of embracing yoga with every ounce of your being—even tolerating you abandoning them carelessly for the comfort only yoga's arms could provide. Yoga was the one-step answer to all of your hot-button issues. You had found your love. But your current state seems so non-namaste that they don't want to play anymore. To them, you've become just another poser.

And now, you're alone, and only one thing rings true:

YOU. Hate. Yoga.

PART 2

YOGA-PHOENIX RISING

Chapter 13

BACK TO THE FUTURE

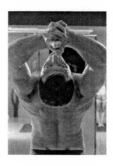

"Healing is a matter of time, but it is sometimes also a matter of opportunity."

—Hippocrates

I n 1995, while performing in a large-scale Toronto production of *Beauty and the Beast*, I started feeling a strange back pain that was causing me significant discomfort, but did not seem to limit my mobility—just a sharp pain at the base of my spine that caused no noticeable physical impairment.

I saw a doctor who sent me for x-rays and a CT scan.

Neither revealed anything. The doctor was a little surprised given the pain I was describing.

I then tried other treatments: Acupuncture, massage therapy, osteopathy. Nothing helped. I still hurt more than a country tune.

Randomly, I ended up in the office of a man by the name of Glenn Boggio. Dr. Boggio is a chiropractor and nutritionist, but those titles—I would later learn—existed only for the sake of medical legitimacy to practice something entirely beyond my comprehension at the time.

His treatments are anything but generic or ordinary in the scope of western medicine—but they worked for me. Within two weeks of seeing Dr. Boggio, my back was feeling better.

It was the first time I had been introduced to the practice of "energy healing."

He didn't do much—small adjustments, yes. He does not adhere to the crack-the-back mentality that other chiropractors stick to.

Mostly, Dr. Boggio just watched.

He watched the energy of my body, and—with his very presence and understanding— adjusted it, balanced it, and got it moving.

I know. You're suddenly kicking yourself for reading this far in what had the potential to be an amusing—perhaps even helpful—book from some Canadian dude with a bit of a 'tude.

But this happened. So stick with me, eh.

On my first visit, I told him that the tests I took showed nothing. He told me they eventually would have. What he was seeing was pain in what was deemed my "energy body." The energy in my base chakra was not moving and the blockage of energy movement was causing me pain. If it continued for much longer, he informed me that it would eventually manifest into the body as something that *could* be diagnosed.

It hadn't gone that far, but he assured me that the pain was real. This I knew.

The science of energy healing is also real but largely controversial with regards to efficacy. If western medicine can't see it, it generally doesn't believe in it.

In 2005, the North American Nursing Diagnosis Association, however, approved "energy field disturbance" in patients as a legitimate diagnosis.

Carolyn Myss is well distinguished as a spiritual healer and intuitive. In her book, *Anatomy of the Spirit*, she explains how energy is a major player in *all* illnesses and presents her "biography becomes biology" doctrine:

> Practitioners of energy medicine believe that the human energy field contains and reflects each individual's energy. It surrounds us and carries with us the emotional energy created by our internal and external experiences—both positive and negative. This emotional force influences the physical tissue within our bodies. In this way, your biography—that is, the experiences that make up your life—becomes your biology.

Her success with patients is well documented and her methods difficult to debate. Put simply, they work through understanding the illnesses not just on a physical level—but an emotional, historical and spiritual level as well.

Learning that the way I process information, experiences and relationships may have been affecting my health, started to bring about an epiphany-like understanding of my ailments, particularly my back pain.

Dr. Boggio helped me with the physical, but the true work would have to come from me or else the pain would rear itself once again, he warned.

But initially—following Boggio's first five treatments—I enjoyed what appeared to be a miraculous turnaround in how I felt. It was a new life. I had been given a golden key, unlocking me from two years of pain-prison.

But then, after a few months, I felt it again.

Back to Boggio.

I told him that it was not the same intensity as before—not even close. But it was there.

Boggio explained that it was going to be my weak area and—while it would never be as potent a pain as before because he had dealt with the initial blockage—it would present itself whenever my energy became imbalanced through emotional turmoil or not living the path I am destined to live.

He was right.

The expression of my creativity became a major theme in the diagnosis and understanding of my back pain.

It came and went—almost predictably so—depending upon the depth of the emotional landscape I pioneered and how I chose to excavate it.

Then came yoga. Yoga, like energy healing, was based on the principle of taking care of the body in order to facilitate the clearing of the mind and potentially open a portal to the human spirit.

Yoga seemed to provide me with further healing, partly due to the innate care of the spine being offered through the Bikram yoga series, but also because the meditative aspect seemed to shut down a lot of what I learned was at the core of my pain: Obsessive thinking!

Chapter 14

I THINK, THEREFORE I'M DAMNED

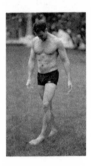

Caught thinking
during a yoga
photo shoot
in the park.

"There is nothing either good or bad, but thinking makes it so."

—William Shakespeare

I n Shakespeare's *Hamlet*, it's argued that the cause for the protagonist's main downfall is the malady of analysis paralysis, or overthinking.

Hamlet is so wrought with thought that it leads to multiple episodes of inaction and— ultimately—his own insanity.

All of Hamlet's joys, instincts and vibrancy of youth are "sicklied over with the pale cast of thought."

Of course, there's also Hamlet's famous "To be or not to be" speech—in which he contemplates suicide—that concludes: "…thus conscience (thinking) does make cowards of us all."

Poor Hamlet. He could have benefited from a lengthy Savasana and a regular yoga practice.

Thinking is entirely overrated. I know this because I do it a lot. But I'm thinking you do, too. The sober truth is that thinking rarely leads to anything resembling greatness.

Great athletes don't think.

In the jaw-dropping autobiography *Open* that details the harrowing career of tennis star Andre Agassi, he credits the art of non-thinking for the reality of winning:

> I can't beat this guy, I know I can't, so I may as well just try to give a good show. Freed from thoughts of winning, I instantly play better. I stop thinking, start feeling. My shots become a half-second quicker, my decisions become the product of instinct rather than logic.

Great artists don't think.

Even great writers steer clear of the thought process; it inevitably produces mediocre results. When artists describe the instruments behind their inspired musings, thinking is rarely given credit.

You don't have to be Einstein to understand this concept, but just in case, let's hear what Albert—labeled one of the great "thinkers" of all time—has to say about his thought process, that he famously described as "muscular."

The words or the language, as they are written or spoken, do not seem to play any role in my mechanism of thought. The psychical entities which seem to serve as elements in thought are certain signs and more or less clear images which can be "voluntarily" reproduced and combined. (Describing his process further): Visual and motor. In a stage when words intervene at all, they are, in my case, purely auditive, but they interfere in a secondary stage.

Put simply, many interpret Einstein's words as meaning that thought is created through feeling and imagery, but actual thinking has very little to do with the process.

The minds of great artists may be used as tools for their work, but it is within the body— the heart—from which the muse manifests and ultimately enables the mind to carry out the technical requirements for completion.

The mind is a much better servant than master.

It serves its purpose, but to credit thought for inspired brilliance would be to place it too high up the brood chain. It's the equivalent of crediting the canvas for the art.

If we think about a tree as we look at it, then we are not really looking at the tree; no evolved, naturally euphoric feeling is accompanied by thought.

In times of great danger—when immediate action is necessary and great rescues are carried out—people never mention "thought" as being a part of the equation because it would simply get in the way of what needed to be done.

The same applies to yoga. Thought only gets in the way of your posture and your progress and, more importantly, the healing potential.

But we are conditioned to think. To validate all of our experiences and feelings, what do we often do? We think about them, thus discrediting their authenticity.

According to a study by *Psychology Today*, approximately 70% of our "mental chatter" is negative, even when those in the study believed the larger percentage of their thoughts to be positive.

The results of the study put all "mental chatter" into three categories:

1. Thoughts related to inferiority
2. Thoughts related to love and approval
3. Thoughts related to control-seeking

I believe that pretty much covers the entire spectrum of our thinking lives, don't you?

The only true solution? Don't think.

There are activities that require or demand—for optimal results—no thinking, or at the very least, work towards shutting down thought. Two such activities would be meditation and yoga. In many respects, they are one in the same.

A *New York Times* article by Oliver Burkeman—which references a 2009 study in *The Journal of Pain*—entitled, "The Power of Negative Thinking," states that even "very brief training in meditation…brought significant reductions in pain—not by ignoring unpleasant sensations, or refusing to feel them, but by turning non-judgmentally toward them."

Yoga does exactly that. It facilitates an active, mindful meditation. Any yoga, whether it is physically demanding or calmly restorative, can help you stop thinking.

Often in a yoga practice—instead of being present with the posture—we begin a dialogue that sabotages the only thing of value: The present moment.

We need to constantly bring ourselves back to the breath, back to the present moment, which, in the words of Eckhart Tolle, is all that ever exists. In his spiritual teachings, he wisely informs us that there are only two things that will never change: Our essence and the present moment.

"It will never not be now," Eckhart writes in his wonderful book, *The Power of Now*.

Luckily, we can release thoughts at any time and bring ourselves back to this moment, the breath and the posture. It is never too late.

But it doesn't start next week or next month. It starts now.

Use your yoga practice as a portal to the human spirit—which is encompassed not by thought, but presence and clarity.

A rigorous hatha yoga series, such as Bikram, puts the body into a state of surrender and submission—a realm from which we can benefit physiologically, energetically and spiritually.

When I started doing yoga and freed myself from the chains of incessant thought, my back pain improved considerably once again.

If you've never practiced yoga, don't *think* about trying it. Just try it.

Leave your brain at the door. You are entering a world of adventure and seemingly unrealistic possibilities brought on by the simple act of doing.

Chapter 15

SEX AND THE PRETTY

"Sex at age ninety is like trying to shoot pool with a rope."

—George Burns

There's a largely unadvertised advantage to having a regular yoga practice.

The sex.

Maybe it's the increased blood flow to the pelvis, the stimulation of the reproductive system or the toning of the sexual core (pelvis and perineum).

I don't know about you, but I'm already craving a cigarette.

Of course it could also be the newly gained confidence that a steady yoga practice can offer, or just the fact that you're getting sweaty, hot and bendy with nimble bodies on numerous occasions, providing fantasy-incentive that can be channeled accordingly.

I'm not sure. (Ahem). Okay, I'm kinda sure.

In the words of one woman to her husband (a client) after he engaged in regular yoga for a few months: "Whatever you're doing, keep doing it."

Let's face it: Yoga's pretty sexy. Students may not be there to hook up, but some of them certainly do.

And, as a bit of a disclaimer, let's get even more real here with my own confession:

I've had sex with people I met or taught at yoga; a few of them even developed into long-term relationships. The sex was always consensual, legal and—more to the point I'd like to emphasize—really damn good!

Yoga people are pretty. Inside and out. I repeat: Inside and out.

The notion that two adults who either work together or share a mature, (adult) student and teacher relationship should not engage in horizontal activity is more antiquated than the idea of creating authentic love through an arranged marriage.

Two adults who decide to get it on are simply two people making a choice—wise or otherwise. Whether the ending plays out as a sweet tune or a shrill squeal is their business. End of story.

Now, let's get back to the sexy stuff.

Whether you are single, married, in an open relationship or a closed one, the sex you and your partner(s) have can be duly enhanced by yoga.

It leaves me curious as to why more men don't practice yoga. Yoga is the natural Viagra—the obvious bonus being that when the sex is over, you don't have to hammer nails with the damn thing in order to exhaust it into submission; another plus being that the long-term effects won't have you growing another one in twenty years.

Yes, I got all recreational (aka stupid) and tried Viagra once in my 30s. Just the memory of the experience makes my little guy retreat like a frightened turtle. We've been at odds about that incident ever since

But that was *before* yoga.

Guys, let's talk man to mini-man here for a moment. Ladies, please jump forward a couple of paragraphs.

Guys. We've all had situations in which we, well, underperformed or, sadly, had to cancel the show all together. These "occurrences" can be humbling and embarrassing, even though it's a known fact that the woman (or man) beside us is usually much more "okay" about it than we are.

We can easily fill up with enough remorse afterward to rival the shame felt by Adam Sandler at the debut of each one of his movies (with the total exception of *Happy Gilmore*).

And while "events" like these do occur with excess alcohol or 4-too-many slices of meat lovers' pizza being just a few likely contributors, we can decrease the odds considerably by practicing yoga just a few times a week. Suddenly, your percentages of winning the "Sex Super Bowl" increase in direct proportion to the non-drug-induced blood flow to your quarterback.

It's a no-brainer. And we like not thinking, don't we guys?

Now, imagine keeping the thinking to a minimum and the blood flow to a maximum well into old age? Yup. Yoga has that capability.

Okay. Good chat. Come on back, ladies.

While yoga for a better sex life simply makes sense, it's probably best not to get too excited and create the expectation of Herculean-like deeds of bravado in the bedroom.

So, let's forget about the flexibility clichés and the feats of endurance that are stereotypically attached to yogis and gymnasts for a moment and focus on something more realistic:

Yoga can increase your flexibility and improve your endurance.

It's all just one happy ending. Then another...and another...

Chapter 16

IT'S A QUIET THING

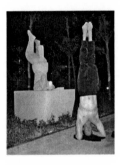

Headstand in
The Mayan Riviera

"The best cure for the body is a quiet mind."
—Napoleon Bonaparte

Having spent most of my life in musical theatre, there are an endless number of songs and lyrics in my head that often come to the surface without warning. Sometimes, they have a serendipitous attachment to the moment and—at other times—they are about as random and inexplicable as a CEO with a nose ring.

Without revealing too much about the peculiar goings-on in my largely uncensored psyche, each time I hear the word "quiet", a Kander and Ebb song lyric always presents itself:

"When it all comes true, just the way you planned, it's funny but the bells don't ring…it's a quiet thing."

The greatest revelations, musings and epiphanies always seem to enter our world through a calm field of quiet.

One of the most joyous aspects of practicing yoga is that once class begins all talking stops. There is no verbal interaction. All personalities (A-Type or otherwise), all social extroverts, all "I love to hear myself talk" folk, must exist within quiet.

This can bring so much discomfort to certain individuals that you're almost sure they'd rather open a vein and die in a pool of their own blood than actually observe silence for an hour or more.

And it's been my observation that it's only getting worse.

In an effort to cater to the decreasing attention span of its listeners, a Calgary radio station (AMP) recently announced that they would only be playing half of each song; and they insist that their new format is here to stay. I assume they feel it's in their best interests to honor the suspected needs of their clientele—even with what would appear to be a backhanded insult to the listeners' intelligence.

Fostering an individual's inability to focus for more than three minutes—as opposed to working on improving their limited concentration skills—isn't likely to help the cause for more quiet time and the healing that comes with it. How can we connect with ourselves in meditation for even 15 minutes if our limited attention spans are not only being appeased but also applauded and rewarded with compliance to the original problem? Why solve the issue when you can just feed it for profit?

If this becomes a trend, the shortened tune could soon become quite a "catchy" metaphor; we will be buying half of a painting because pondering and reflecting the entire work would just be too overwhelming and time-consuming. Or even worse, we will begin to recognize only half of our feelings because delving into the whole heart will seem inconvenient and futile.

If you think that sounds silly, take yourself back 10 years and try to imagine a radio station playing only half of each artist's song. Anarchy would follow, whereas today it conjures up only half the ire it actually warrants. Fitting, I suppose.

The proliferation of gadgets, games and gizmos that cater to (and actually encourage) instant gratification—along with an attention span so short it barely even starts—is creating a world in which the act of internalizing is becoming as ancient as the first iPhone.

Quieting the mind, the mouth, and going on a journey inward is not only a lofty goal, it's a daunting one.

It's possible that people have never been more afraid of quiet.

Yet, we need it more than ever. The brain buzzing is moving us further away from an understanding of the body, the mind and all of the beautifully subtle distinctions that can be made with regards to our physical, mental and emotional makeup.

A yoga practice is a great place to start.

As the body expresses itself with each posture and the continuous work to shut down the brain ensues, the potential discoveries can be so profound that one may wish to shout to the heavens and share the moment; but there is so much reward in the continuity and integrity of quiet that breaking the seal will not even be an option.

It's like finding a secret tree as a child—one that only you climb and inhabit. You don't dare tell anyone.

In the thoughtful book *Quiet* by Susan Cain, she gives astute merit to introversion and its somewhat unheralded strengths:

> Whoever you are, bear in mind that appearance is not reality. Some people act like extroverts, but the effort costs them energy, authenticity, and even physical health. Others seem aloof or self-contained, but their inner landscapes are rich and full of drama. So the next time you see a person with a composed face and a soft voice, remember that inside her mind she might be solving an equation, composing a sonnet, designing a hat. She might, that is, be deploying the powers of quiet.

Use the silent state of a yoga practice to carve away the world's distractions and present you with the glorious gift of authenticity and an *entire* tune worth singing:

"When it all comes true...the bells don't ring..."

"It's a quiet thing."

Chapter 17

A PINCH OF HEAVEN,
A CUP OF HELL

Ego says, "Once everything falls into place, I will find peace." Spirit says, "Find your peace and everything will fall into place."

—Marianne Williamson

Have you ever heard the story about the samurai who sought out the true nature of heaven and hell?

The brave warrior, in an attempt to gain wisdom and insight, searched for this meaning for much of his life.

He spent years sailing across tumultuous seas, scaling angry mountains, occupying countless Starbucks outlets and asking everyone he encountered if they knew where he could attain this knowledge—which he felt to be one of the key ingredients to eternal happiness.

After an extensive, thorough journey, he was bereft.

There was only one village he had not visited.

As luck would have it, the people of the village informed the weary samurai that they knew where he could find his answer.

There was a wise man that lived alone atop the mountain on the edge of the village. If the samurai made the journey, he would most certainly be awarded this secret and thus be spiritually fulfilled.

It was one of the most daunting mountains he had ever seen, but he had come this far, so he courageously began his purposeful expedition.

His sheer will carried him up the mountain and, finally, he stood before the wise man who was said to possess the elusive wisdom he coveted.

"I have traveled my whole life for this moment," he anxiously told the wise man. "I have been told that you understand the true nature of heaven and hell. Can you please share this wisdom with me?"

The wise man looked the samurai up and down and, with unrelenting fervor, suddenly began spewing venomous rhetoric towards the shell-shocked warrior:

"Why would I share such information with a ridiculous character such as yourself? How stupidly presumptuous and foolhardy you must be to think that someone with my stature would offer up such valuable wisdom to a stupid lowlife like you!"

The wise man continued to stab the warrior with dagger-like insults for what seemed to be hours and, all the while, the samurai's rage was igniting like a fuel-soaked bonfire.

Finally, it was too much to take. The samurai drew his sword, held it high in the air and was a moment away from cutting off the head of the supposed wise man—who continued to feverishly belittle him and his life-long quest for the true nature of heaven and hell.

Just as the blade was to sever the head of the wise man, he looked deep into the eyes of the angered warrior and spoke with calm, knowing clarity:

"That's hell," he said.

Upon hearing these words, the samurai slowly put down his sword, sat down on a rock and began to weep. He realized with sadness that he had let the wise man provoke him into a fiery dance with his own ego—the result of which would have been tragic.

As he continued to weep in shame, the wise man walked over to him, gently put his hand on his shoulder and said compassionately, "That's heaven."

This has always been a beautifully penetrating story for me because I believe there is no better tale to describe how we create our own heaven and hell.

Unfortunately, it is often easier to construct our own hell in any situation that presents adversity because it is the easier way out every time. Staying in that hell seems like a safe choice to many. We can choose anger over deep contemplation and sadness, yet, scratch the surface of anger, and you will find sadness almost every time.

On several occasions—with yoga as their conduit—I've seen individuals come face-to-face with momentous growth only to succumb to a daunting feeling of hardship and quickly abandon their journey before it truly starts to benefit them.

It's a frustrating scene to witness. A single soul—just weeks or even days away from making significant progress—looks up the mountain they have begun to climb, then quickly turns and begins to walk back down.

"The weather got too rough," they'd say. "I'll try again next week."

But they rarely do.

In the yoga world, the excuses are usually predictable: "I just stopped having the time." "I don't deal well with the heat." "I didn't like the teacher."

We can talk ourselves out of anything—even a yoga practice that can prove to be of immense benefit to our well-being. Some are ready to break out of old patterns and comfortable habits to bravely embrace the next chapter, and some simply are not.

One of the gifts of owning a yoga studio is that sometimes a person walks in—having never done yoga—and stands in front of you with a vulnerability so pure you would only witness it on the face of a newborn baby.

They don't even know why they're there. They just know that something's gotta give with the life they've been leading. A courageous voice in their body brought them to a yoga studio.

Their expression speaks to something deeper than a simple conscious choice to start a yoga practice. It's tough to give it a word description without stripping it of its spiritual potency, except to say that the energy surrounding the moment is as raw, real and beautiful as that of anything I have ever felt.

They're ready. For something. Anything.

There is another story I once heard from Eckhart Tolle about a man who is considering moving to a new town. He goes into the local café and talks to a regular patron: "I'm thinking of moving to your town. What are the people like?"

The local answers with his own question: "What are the people like in the town you just came from?"

"Oh, they are awful people. Very deceitful, unkind and unfriendly," the man spews without hesitation.

The local citizen quips: "Well, I think you'll find they're much the same here."

Months later, another man enters the café with the same inquiry and wanders up to the same regular.

"I'm thinking of moving to your town. What are the people like here?"

Again, he answers with the same degree of curiosity: "Well, what are they like in the town you just came from?"

"Wonderful. They are lovely, kind, gentle and giving," the man says with a fond smile.

"Well, I think you will find they are much the same here," the local offers back.

We have to take responsibility for our happiness. We are not entitled to it and our perceptions can be the game-changer.

Yoga can be a signpost on your journey, but if you don't try it, you'll never know if it's a step in the right direction.

A yoga journey can be difficult, but it can also be endlessly rewarding and, who knows, the true nature of heaven and hell—as it pertains to you personally—may be revealed along the way.

Chapter 18

COLOR ME YOGA

"If we cannot end now our differences, at least we can help make the world safe for diversity. For, in the final analysis, our most basic common link is that we all inhabit this small planet."
—John F. Kennedy *[Commencement Address at American University, June 10, 1963]*

'm proud to say, as a long-time Torontonian, that Toronto holds the distinction of being one of the most culturally diverse cities in the world. Almost half of Toronto's population is comprised of visible minorities and—unlike other diverse cities—its foreign-born population is not dominated by any particular ethnic group.

There is no better visual example of this than in a Toronto yoga class.

But what makes the energy of a room filled with individuals of varied cultural backgrounds even more beautifully potent is the complete lack of exclusivity in the air.

Yoga is not elite or discriminatory. It's accessible. To everyone.

Catholics go to church with other Catholics. Professional athletes belong to an exclusive club based on their abilities and gender; even amateur sports have standards and conditions that must be met before joining. Democrats are generally not welcome at a Republican convention and vegans are often looked upon with disdain in a meat-loving household.

There are no such restrictions or judgments in yoga—and that extends to your physicality and health.

There is no measure of your flexibility or strength before you walk into a yoga room; you practice yoga to *become* strong and flexible. You also practice to heal, and that healing looks different for everyone.

Some students of yoga are there to help them get through a break-up—others for back problems or knee issues or to recover from a car accident. They may wish to lower their blood pressure, lose some weight, quiet their mind, relieve depression, or even recover from cancer, but none of these issues carry the tag of being a prerequisite in order to "belong."

Everyone belongs—the ill, the healthy, the Protestants, the Jews, the opinionated, the silly, the eccentric and the socially-awkward.

In fact, I have students who I know love coming to yoga simply because they feel welcome in the studio, free from all the demands and social standards of the outside world. Ironically, the yoga and its benefits are secondary to the untainted solace they feel in a yoga environment in which they are made to feel safe and accepted. There are no "club criteria" or labels that may be attached to being a member of the math, chess or debating club. The criteria are simple: Get on your mat and discover you.

Some may argue that the "financially-challenged" are limited in their quest to be a yogi, given the cost of maintaining a regular yoga practice. But if you consider the fact that most studios offer up a "trade" or "energy exchange" program in which free yoga is exchanged for a mere few hours of work per week at the studio, this line of reasoning is quickly defused.

We have over 25 individuals enrolled in our energy exchange program at my studio. It benefits both parties and lends to our vision statement that is based on a simple theory: More people doing yoga benefits everyone.

It's a domino effect in which personal health can only translate into more energy, which culminates into better productivity, greater self-worth, more awareness and a clearer perspective on issues such as, well, discrimination and exclusivity in the world.

It's the circle of life, Simba.

In a world in which racism remains abhorrently prevalent, yoga—by its very definition of "union"—facilitates diversity by shrugging its shoulders at the notion that it might actually matter what color you are or what belief system you adhere to in order to benefit fully from a yoga practice.

The very thought doesn't even deserve the energy it might take to consider it.

In an earlier chapter, I stated that religion and yoga don't mix and I stand by that, but let's make it clear that those who choose religion usually don't practice their religion in the yoga room.

They practice yoga.

They also don't speak of political beliefs or sexual preferences. Generally, they don't speak at all because they are there to connect with the unbiased essence of their body and spirit.

Yoga exists to strip us of our labels, not propagate them.

There is a commonality amongst yogis of every age, shape and background that exists when the yoga train is boarded: Acceptance.

This presents an interesting reality:

The only thing that can really keep you from doing yoga… is you.

Chapter 19

"TAKE TWO AND CALL ME WITH A WARNING"

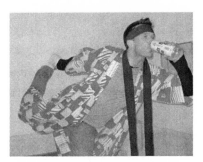

Finding "balance"
during a trip to Japan

"One of the first duties of the physician is to educate the masses not to take medicine."

—William Oslerd

It's of merit to note that the medical benefits of a yoga practice can, potentially, keep you from having to see a physician, which ultimately may keep you away from something much more damaging than a yoga teacher who likes playing doctor: Prescription drugs.

Earlier, we destroyed the idea of a yoga-doctor. Now, let's take a look at some statistics and entertain the possibility that, while your teacher may not be a doctor, a yoga practice may be safer than what your doctor is doling out.

I once heard it said that "Western medicine uses a canon to kill a mosquito" and I couldn't agree more.

The side effects of prescription drugs and their ability to hide symptoms without touching on the real problem are adding layers upon layers of issues that go beyond just the physical. Instead of moving closer to understanding your body by balancing its energy and makeup, these drugs create numbness—and the possibility of an emotional imbalance that could have damaging effects, not just to the person taking them, but to others as well.

Many prescription drugs save lives. That is a wonderful reality. But they also move people further away from their essence—and an astute understanding of their bodies and minds.

They also lead to addiction.

The Center for Disease Control and Prevention reports that, in the decade leading up to 2007, the percentage of Americans who took at least one prescription drug in the past month increased by 10%. The use of multiple prescription drugs increased by 20% and the use of five or more drugs increased by 70%. By 2007-2008, one half of Americans used at least one or more prescription drugs—and one out of 10 used five or more. One out of every five children used at least one or more prescription drugs compared with nine of every 10 adults aged 60 and over.

This is a distressing trend towards overuse and abuse leading to premature death, and studies are showing that it's getting alarmingly worse:

According to the United States Department of Health and Human Services, drug overdose death rates have increased five-fold since 1980. By 2009, drug overdose deaths outnumbered deaths due to motor vehicle crashes for the first time in U.S. history, and prescription drugs have been increasingly involved in drug overdose deaths.

Again, there is a place for prescription drugs, but the disturbing development with humankind is that we tend to take things to extremes. We are already doing so at the expense of our environment—with no end in sight to the damage we will inflict upon generations to follow.

It should come as no surprise that we're overusing prescription drugs.

The strange mindset seems to be that if there's a pill for what ails us, it only makes sense to swallow it, but we know where that reasoning leads us. The damage we may be causing ourselves is an even tougher pill to swallow.

It's an interesting irony that prescription drugs can help us live longer, but at the possible expense of our quality of life. There is more chronic pain and disease than ever. The true problems are not being tackled, the symptoms are.

There are many cautionary tales regarding the use of prescription drugs and while mine may not be the most thrilling, it serves the purpose.

I have always had problems with sleeping. Years before I discovered yoga, I remember going to my doctor to discuss the matter. I explained that I never have issues with getting to sleep, just waking up in the middle of the night and not being able to get back to sleep for hours. As a music theatre performer, this was becoming an issue because sleep was essential for my vocal stamina.

The doctor listened, and then wrote me a prescription for a sleep medication.

They were great. Problem solved. I was sleeping like a baby minus the wetting and wailing.

Back then I didn't realize there would be side effects or long-term implications because I was not warned of any. I was an impressionable lad in my 20s who just needed to get some sleep in order to perform at an optimal level on stage.

I do remember being told that they were "habit-forming" but so is making the bed every morning. The word "addictive" was not used and, as I said earlier here, my exposure to addiction awakens precautions in me that others may not need to exercise.

When I started to understand—through my own research—the implications of the choice I was making in taking these pills, I decided to get off of them, but it was a little too late. I was hooked. I panicked and quit cold turkey, which of course caused endless nights of no sleep and more anxiety than I started with.

Years later, I would discover yoga and, while sleep and I still (on occasion) don't share the same bed, I now enjoy healthy amounts of shut-eye. Yoga helped me immensely.

Yes, I still take the occasional sleeping pill, but that's because, every now and then, I succumb to the quick fix that is accessible to me. I don't *need* to. But I do.

This might be a good time to mention that perfection has never been on my bucket list. I practice yoga, not perfection. It's all a work in progress, and yoga helps me put my gloves on when a fight with temptation is imminent.

But when I think back to the power of the doctor in front me during that initial sleep-concerned visit, I want to rewrite the "script" and have him hand me a piece of paper with two words on it: Try yoga.

Your yoga teacher isn't your doctor, but yoga as a prescription for overall health just might be the best advice any doctor could give you—and such advice is becoming increasingly popular:

A Harvard University study published in May of 2013 found that more than 6.3 million Americans use mind-body therapies—including yoga and meditation—based on a referral from their physicians.

A combination of doctors prescribing yoga and good instructors teaching it could be the most powerful hybrid for health yet.

The prudent distinction between the two, however, must also be prescribed.

Chapter 20

TWISTED TERROR

"We fear things in proportion to our ignorance of them."
—Christian Nestell Bovee

Yoga can be used as a tool to alleviate anxiety and fear. But when the fear is the yoga itself, a powerful practice for healing suddenly becomes part of the problem, not the solution.

How can the very thing that may *heal* your fears *be* your fear? How do we go on a mind-twisting, backwards journey that begins with "yoga will ease my fears" to "I'm afraid of yoga?"

It's a path easily taken.

I often have students, who are about to take their first class, approach the desk and disclose with no amount of hesitation that they are afraid. They have heard horror stories of students passing out, vomiting and struggling for breath.

The stories are true.

It doesn't happen often, but a number of factors can contribute to such an event. Usually, it's a simple hydration issue, but frequently they are actually being given a gift in the form of a diagnosis. Yoga can be a great diagnostic tool, revealing underlying issues that are brought up, often unpleasantly, as you explore your body.

From an emotional perspective, we usually have to fully feel something before we can fully let it go.

But people don't die during yoga or because of it. There are so many precautions around hot yoga in particular, and they are usually over-dramatized by those who have never tried it.

But let's step back for a moment. For whatever reason, the student is legitimately afraid. Of yoga.

It's an honest admission and, given the history and reputation built around Bikram yoga in particular, it's also an accurate, understandable feeling.

Yet, there they are—at a yoga studio. They have come to yoga despite the fear-factor because they have also been told of the health benefits, and the feeling of elation and clarity following a class.

As I pointed out earlier, Bikram yoga has built up, through its own devices, a reputation for being "survival yoga" of the hardcore nature for A-Type personalities.

While many are aware of its beneficial properties, I suspect even more remain terrified of trying it, and adding more layers of fear with militant teaching methods certainly doesn't help.

Many new students enter the yoga studio carrying with them the debilitating characteristics of shyness, insecurity and poor self-value. Is being tough on them out of the gate going to set the platform for safe healing and enable them to do their very best?

There is another way—a way that removes the dread and makes this largely accessible yoga even more accessible with the realization that there is *nothing* to fear. It will still be hard work, but that reality will not be pre-empted by fear.

It all has to do with the environment created by each studio for each student walking in the door to the yoga studio. A safe, kind environment in which to accommodate healing is the only formula I can endorse. I also argue that it's the only one that works.

Intimidation and fear tactics in yoga are as ridiculously ineffective and convoluted as believing you need to have a fear of flying in order to become a good pilot.

There are no studies that show that people become great yogis when taught under a blanket of fear and there's a simple reason for that: It would be entertaining a notion that goes against every grain of common sense.

But there *are* studies that prove that using fear as a motivator not only doesn't produce the desired results, it actually can make matters worse.

Psychcentral.com covered a controlled study for many years:

Scared Straight was a program designed to deter juveniles from criminal offenses. Participants have interaction with adult inmates through visitations so that they can observe prison life first-hand. These programs are common in many areas of the world.

The simple principle of these programs are that juveniles who see what prison is like will be dissuaded from future violations of the law—in other words, "scared straight."

The problem is, it backfired:

One analysis showed *Scared Straight* interventions could possibly worsen conduct-disorder symptoms and another showed that *Scared Straight* and similar programs produced substantial increases in recidivism (chronic relapse into crime).

The evidence concluded that *Scared Straight* and similar programs are not effective in deterring criminal activity in the youths participating. Conversely, it was concluded that these types of programs might just be harmful and increase delinquency compared to no intervention at all with the same participants.

Implementing fear as a tactic for rehabilitation or healing is simply an archaic principle and can only lead to hardening the heart and depleting the soul, the manifesting of more fear and thus, more problems.

Another branch on the tree of yoga fear would be that of ego, and its buds are largely male.

A 2012 survey by Yoga Journal found that of the 20.4 million people who practice yoga in the United States, only 18% of them are men.

It's been well documented, through thousands of years of killing each other, that men possess the ego-gene and wear it mistakenly as healthy pride.

I can tell you from experience that a man's displeasure in the possibility of performing poorly does not facilitate the yoga adventure.

Instilling a "fear-factor" upon yoga only triggers yet another leg of fear: The fear of failure. It's a double whammy of intimidation.

Men are more prey to this formula.

Regardless of gender, your yoga practice is a subjective journey and—as you embark upon that exploration of body, mind and spirit through physical practice—it's essential that fear, intimidation, competition, performance, ego and grandstanding in the form of entitlement and expectation be obliterated from the landscape.

Be not afraid of yoga.

Learning how to swim may present some difficulties if you're convinced you have a fear of water.

The best strategy might just be to jump right in.

Chapter 21

FASHION A FEELING?

"The most beautiful makeup of a woman is passion. But cosmetics are easier to buy."
—Yves Saint-Laurent

n 2013, I went to see my first runway fashion show during Toronto Fashion Week.

I had never been to a fashion show and I was curious. I wanted to experience this world that, from what I could gather, was built on a foundation of image—and how tall pretty women look in different items of clothing.

I didn't see any harm in it. Like most men with a pulse, I am not immune to the enjoyment of watching crazily attractive females walk around in sexy clothing. And while being handed a license to do so under the guise of "art" seemed like a bit of a game to me, it was a game I was willing to engage in for the evening. Hedonism is alive and well in my soul—in what I deem to be healthy increments.

What I experienced was surprising. I shouldn't have expected more than what I, well, expected.

The overly-amplified music kicked in and, one-by-one, the models strutted briskly down the catwalk, expressionless. For a moment, I imagined that they had been programmed in some way, chips inserted into their brains, triggering an explosion if a thought even had the potential to produce one readable emotion on their faces.

While everyone around me seemed to be fully engaged in the proceedings, I was stunned by how eerily detached the models seemed to be, not just from their hip joints, but their surroundings.

I had a strange urge to yell out at one to see if I could provoke a reaction.

I wanted connection.

I felt like a desperate partner being dumped, screaming out for validation and acceptance. Needy. I felt needy—wanting more milk from a dried-up udder.

It wasn't enough for me that they were beautiful women in clean clothes. In retrospect, I guess it should have been.

It reminded me of the advice I give my teachers when they get physically or verbally lazy with their instruction: "Hey, if you're not engaged, why should we be? You need to ignite inspiration, not expect it."

But then I realized something somewhat profound—which would seem odd given my surroundings.

I realized that this was all *my* fault. You see, I was focusing on the women when clearly the main point of interest was supposed to be the designer's clothing.

I forgot what it was about. It was about the designer and the clothing. Not the women. Duh! They were there to serve the clothing and that's what they were doing—their jobs.

They didn't have to care about me. And they didn't.

I didn't have to care about them. But I did.

I was wrong. They were right.

Besides being arguably undernourished, they seemed fine with it all. Their modus operandi was simple: Strut without falling. There was nothing in the model manual about energy and caring.

The fact that I wanted more was clearly *my* issue, not theirs. I've always been more comfortable in surroundings where people are connecting in some way and I can feel the exchange of energy, not its polarization.

So, all this to say that—to no fault of anyone but my own—I didn't like the fashion show. It seemed to lack heart to me. Pretty without heart has its place, I suppose, and that evening I thought it would suffice, but it obviously revealed a chasm of discomfort in me that I wouldn't want to revisit.

As I was leaving the fashion show, the importance of connection struck me harder than a stiletto on the catwalk.

It's my observation that there is too much numbness in the world, and its proliferation is only accentuated by disengaged events like that of models coming off as soulless while promoting clothing.

Again, I obviously missed the point. I suppose there's a place for it. Why not?

But in writing a book about yoga and how I believe it can awaken individuals by steering them towards health and lucidity, my experience at the fashion show tells me that perhaps we're giving too much attention to the wrong platforms.

Surely, if there is time to be stimulated visually by designer clothing on women *pretending* to be vapid—it would be destructively cliché and entirely untrue to generalize that *all* models are void of emotional depth—there is even *more* time and energy to turn the attention inward, connect with one's self and enjoy greater dividends by doing so.

It's time well spent.

Again, I like to look at pretty things—I'm guessing most of us do—but if we prioritize such activities and give them too much weight in our lives, we might just forget to turn the camera inward and explore the unique beauty that exists within each of us.

Not all yoga is practiced in front of mirrors but Bikram yoga is and I will share the following from experience: When you are about to begin your practice and you stand in front of that mirror—staring into the eyes of the one person you spend the most time with—and you learn to like what you see, you can enter into a world so beautiful that accoutrements of any kind will only take away from the authenticity of the connection established; a connection that could be the beginning of a profoundly healing, loving liaison.

Yoga can help facilitate such a relationship.

What could be more in fashion?

Chapter 22

YOGA'S NOT BORING, YOU ARE!

"The only horrible thing in the world is ennui, Dorian. That is the one sin for which there is no forgiveness."
—from "The Picture of Dorian Gray", by Oscar Wilde

There is no such thing as boredom, only people choosing to be bored. When I—somewhat cheekily—exclaim to students in classes I teach that "the yoga's not boring, *you* are," I often don't get the opportunity to explain further. I am not judging anyone. I'm telling students that they're better than the boredom copout.

Boredom is an easy way out because it relieves us of accountability and responsibility. It enables us to bask in a self-imposed passiveness that is the antithesis of creativity and curiosity.

There is no good that will come from succumbing to what we might feel to be boredom.

It's noteworthy that the word boredom only came into existence about 160 years ago in a Dickens novel, not long after the beginning of the industrial revolution.

I'm going to take the liberty of surmising that, before then, people just didn't have the damn time to be bored. This is why the word only came into being once machines allowed us to kick up our feet and quickly create problems that once didn't exist—boredom being one of them.

In yoga, boredom could be synonymous with not being present or mindful, and both of these states can lead to injury if chosen while in the middle of a posture. I've seen minds wander aimlessly in class with self-made boredom leading the tour and, seconds later, I witness an injury. I can count on one hand the number of times it's happened, but strangely enough, it's always been a student who has been practicing for years; someone whose familiarity of the postures becomes a liability once the link of body and mind are even momentarily lost.

Our minds are busier than ever these days, and we are so used to constant stimulation that a dip in the exhilaration monitor can make us feel like we're about to flatline, when it may just be an opportunity for invaluable self-awareness.

Shutting down the mind can lead to blissful euphoria as you explore an astute connection with your body. There is nothing boring about such an exploration, but self-motivation has to be given value here.

Sometimes, it's simply a matter of redefining our feeling. What if "feeling bored" could be changed into the phrase, "not feeling self-motivated?" Okay, now the onus to change the feeling is on *you*, as opposed to allowing yourself to be a victim of the term boredom.

It's a start.

Then take it further and ask yourself this: What thoughts am I allowing to manifest that are enabling me to feel this way, and if you prescribe to the credo that "our thoughts create our feelings," then the solution is simple: Change the thought; change the feeling.

But prying yourself out of the stigma of boredom is only beneficial if you choose to acknowledge the feeling, see it as unproductive and—like an emotional alchemist—create a positive potion for change.

It's an active transformation. Remember, the only way out is through.

A conclusive study was done in which a theory was supported that pathological gamblers seek stimulation to avoid states of boredom and depression for fear of them; just another example of the fact that we need to acknowledge and honor all of our feelings *before* letting them go—even boredom.

But if the feelings don't serve us, what's the point of hanging out with them too long? This is where boredom and depression become bedmates. Spend too much time languishing in what you feel to be "boredom" and suddenly depression may invite itself in to join the solo pity-party.

Once again, acknowledge the feeling, identify it as something that doesn't serve you and let it go. Easier said than done, I know, but having a formula can often be empowering.

A yoga practice is an exploration of mind, body and spirit. Whether you are just beginning, about to begin, or have been practicing for years, each moment presents you with a choice:

You can either choose to be an adventurer and delve into the unique subtleties of your body as it facilitates and embraces change, or you can fall prey to a feeling you largely manufacture (boredom) and bask in the dim light of mediocrity— illuminated by boredom and shadowed by depression.

I have no problem admitting that I have yet to figure out the endless complexities of each and every posture in the Hatha yoga series and, last time I checked, I owned a yoga studio.

But if I felt I knew all there was to know, my adventure would be over, and then so would my yoga practice and all the health benefits that go with it.

It's a simple fact that children are much easier to teach than adults because they already know that they don't know. Adults sometimes embody a conceit that prohibits progress, protects the ego and ultimately stifles learning.

But there is an easy fix when it comes to yoga.

It's called "beginner's mind." Each and every time you start your practice, pay attention to each detail of form as though you were learning it for the first time. Be explorative, adventurous and curious.

Eliminate the word "boredom" from your vocabulary, your life and your yoga.

Instead, let's stand face-to-face with the fiery essence of adversity and change. In other words, get interested.

The excitement will be tangible.

Chapter 23

BALANCE, MODERATION AND OTHER EXTREMES

"Time and balance are the two most difficult things to have control over, yet they are both the things that we do control."

—Catherine Pulsifer

B alance is a subjective word.

One person's extremes can be seen as another individual's way of achieving equilibrium.

Some of us are instinctively gifted when it comes to bringing balance to our lives. For others, it takes an illness or disease—an extreme—to create balance.

I once interviewed the former CEO of TD Bank, Peter Godsoe. I was writing his bio for a special presentation that would induct him into The Canadian Business Hall of Fame.

He was a fascinating, calm, kind man who attributed his success to one word: Balance.

This is a man whose professional responsibilities, no doubt, carried great weight; but he didn't see it that way.

Yes, he exuded confidence with regards to his vocation, but when he spoke of his time as CEO, he did so only with joy; no drama or burdensome pressure accompanied his speech. He worked hard, yes, but he also spent valuable time with his family, stayed physically active, traveled, enjoyed friends and many other interests which contributed to his "balance" philosophy.

Embracing his family enabled him to fully embrace his work and vice versa. He gave fully to all that was in front of him and never too much to one thing. He didn't get caught up in "overworked" clichés as much as he accepted his work and found pleasure in it because it was one part of a balanced landscape.

The simplicity with which he spoke of this balance was marvelous to me because he made it sound so elementary.

There was nothing self-righteous or forcibly prescribed about his doctrine, but I did get the sense that the underlying message was that balance is not only a necessary ingredient for personal and professional success, but integral to navigating us through the maze toward health and happiness.

I once heard spiritualist and motivational speaker Wayne Dyer say, "Of the hundreds of death-bed regrets I have ever heard, not one of them was, 'I wish I'd spent more time at the office'."

There are some of you who will read this and think that—being a guy who owns a yoga studio—I don't understand the pressure of the western work world, including the uncompromising demands placed on some of you involved with ruthless corporations, but I instinctively feel as though I do, if only by association. It's all relative.

I talk with my yoga students about their work burdens every day, and as the owner of a small business, I am not immune to any of these conditions—the obvious difference being that, for me, they are often self-imposed. I offer up to you, for your mature consideration, that to a large degree, *yours* are also self-imposed.

Different formula. Same nightmare.

My point is this: I discuss with individuals the great stress that their job brings, but that stress also brings many of them to yoga.

That's balance.

I have great respect for those who are clear that, "Yoga doesn't take time. It gives time,"— time to bask in the lucidity of a balanced life.

Stress is often present in at least one aspect of our lives and yoga can ease that stress, offering perspective and calmness. Again, that is balance.

Epictetus said, "If one oversteps the bounds of moderation, the greatest pleasures cease to please."

So, how much work? How much yoga? How much chocolate? That's up to you. But a happy, healthy balance is most certainly available to all of us. The first step is to choose it. How? One way would be to trust your instincts.

Hey, let's face it; we all know when we're crossing the moral line in the sand that our instincts draw out for us so clearly. We just choose not to listen or we internally rationalize our choice, fooling no one but ourselves.

Being honest with ourselves can then be the catalyst that sparks the balance needed, but be careful. Honesty should always be accompanied by responsibility. We've all seen honesty quickly morph into brutal, unnecessary truth. It's a quick and unadvised leap.

I've seen this first-hand as a student who suddenly feels they have a new yoga-lease on life, loses all inhibitions—and with them, common decency—as they verbally cut up everyone in their path with their self-righteous truth sword. It's a bloody scene, usually made bloodier when capped off with the words, "Well, I was only being honest."

Even something as seemingly simple and noble as truth can learn from the ever-changing—and perhaps less smug— moniker of balance.

There is so much to navigate in this crazy, wonderful world, and as we embark on each of our uniquely subjective journeys, yoga can help us to read our compass a little easier, often steering us into choppy waters and fierce winds, yes, but both being beautifully tempered by the strong sails of balance.

Chapter 24

"I'M SORRY, I'M JUST NOT THAT INTUIT-IVE."

"There can be as much value in the blink of an eye as in months of rational analysis."
—Malcolm Gladwell, *Blink: The Power of Thinking Without Thinking*

In the words of medical intuitive and spiritual teacher, Carolyn Myss, intuition is "the voice of your conscience… your gut instinct. It's the voice you don't want to hear, that never turns off."

During an interview with Oprah Winfrey, she muses, "We have an intuitive voice in all of us. We are born intuitive. We are so intuitive that it's actually, for the most part, the source of (our) greatest suffering."

Oprah, perplexed, inquires as to how it could be possible that our intuition might cause us such suffering, and Myss responds prophetically:

"Because people hear when they betray themselves."

We have all participated in this form of self-punishment—not taking action because the action has uncomfortable consequences—only to chastise ourselves for not doing what we know to be right.

We take too long to get out of relationships that no longer fulfill us, or we stay stuck in dead-end, thankless jobs for fear of losing security and regular income.

We do our best to bask in the dim—but sustainable—glow of "normality" because the alternative is just too painful; we ignore all instincts and succumb to the semi-catatonic state of feeling "comfortably numb."

It's truly no way to live.

But what if there was a vehicle for change that could lead us to the necessary action we already instinctively know to be necessary? What if there was a tool in the box that slowly unhinged the weighty door of inner confinement to reveal a courageous path of uncompromising genuineness?

Good news. There is. It's called yoga.

A yoga practice can help put a focus on that which you have been avoiding. It can enable you to trust your instincts and gain the courage to act on them through the simple practice of awareness and acceptance. Yoga can be that missing ingredient that enables you to spice up your recipe for empowerment.

Incremental change is usually imminent. It may not be profound, but it may be just enough to push you in the direction of finally listening to your instincts. Unlike the transparent, pseudo-transformations mentioned in a previous chapter, I've seen it happen authentically right before my eyes.

It often isn't pretty, but it's beautifully liberating.

There are many examples of yoga students gaining the confidence to finally take the steps to change by removing aspects of their life that no longer serve them. The change takes on many forms—not just the obvious chestnut of buying a one-way ticket to India or Indonesia.

But hey, whatever works. If a location has resonated deeply for years, it may just be a sign. As the spiritual credo goes, "Listen to the whispers."

But how can yoga lead someone on a path to his or her holy grail? It's simple.

There is an awakening through the exploration of the body and the calming of the mind that a simple yoga practice can offer. In such a journey, confidence and faith are cultivated and change doesn't seem so difficult.

On the contrary, it usually seems necessary.

Without delving into the useless realm of regret, I have to say that I wish I had trusted my instincts during college—and at other unmentioned times during my life—instead of abandoning them for the cloudy principles of others and, in retrospect, the misty realm of lower ground.

My bad.

But it's never too late. As I stated earlier, yoga ended up helping with my ability to embrace my uniqueness, and rise up on the shoulders of intuition. It can help you, too.

A study on the value of trusting your instincts and its findings was published in the journal, *Proceedings of the National Academy of Sciences* in 2012.

Forced to choose between two options based on instinct alone, participants made the right call up to 90% of the time.

Professor Marius Usher of Tel Aviv University's School of Psychological Sciences and his fellow researchers say their findings reveal that intuition was a surprisingly powerful and accurate tool.

The story, reported in London's *Daily Mail*, details the experiment:

> On a computer screen, participants were shown sequences of pairs of numbers in quick succession. All numbers that appeared on the right of the screen and all on the left were considered a group; each group represented returns on the stock market.
>
> Participants were asked to choose which of the two groups of numbers had the highest average.
>
> Because the numbers changed so quickly—two to four pairs every second—the participants were unable to memorize the numbers or do proper mathematical calculations. To determine the highest average of either group, they had to rely on intuitive arithmetic.
>
> Their accuracy increased when more data was presented.

When shown six pairs of numbers the participants chose accurately 65% of the time. But when they were shown 24 pairs, the accuracy rate grew to about 90%.

"Intuitively, the human brain has the capacity to take in many pieces of information and decide on an overall value," said Professor Usher.

"Gut reactions can be trusted to make a quality decision."

The instincts you can foster and learn to trust through yoga can bring you closer to living a life that feels genuine for you.

What yoga *won't* do for you is make you perfect. It will provide you with a much more valuable spiritual asset than perfection: Acceptance.

Chapter 25

YOGA'S FUNNY
AND SO ARE YOU!

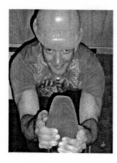

Backstage during a
production of
The Buddy Holly Story

*"My method is to take the utmost trouble to find the right
thing to say, and then to say it with the utmost levity."*
—George Bernard Shaw

Yoga can be serious business.

Sweating out whatever ails ya can often be a harrowing journey through the elusive trifecta of mind, body and spirit; the emotional tools you decide to take with you on this (sometimes daunting) exploration, can be the difference between embracing your practice or simply tolerating it.

Part of the answer to opening your body up sufficiently and maintaining a purposeful focus comes from allowing the all-too-neglected ingredient of levity into your yoga zone.

While in the middle of a posture, you can stare in the mirror and realize that your face has never looked so tight or intense. It's as if you're in the middle of a debilitating brain-freeze from drinking a frozen smoothie too quickly.

This intensity, in the form of energy, manifests into your body creating even more tension and suddenly all your yogi friends have a new nickname for you: SKY!

Serial. Killer. Yogi. An unwelcoming endearment bestowed upon you in an effort to get you to LIGHTEN THE HELL UP.

Yoga can be innately difficult and it needs to be balanced with the joyous infusion of levity.

When I joke in class, it is never with the intention of having students lose their focus. The goal is to actually get them to increase it. Perspective can do just that. After an infusion of humor, the body opens up and the next posture is embraced with lighthearted joy.

Ever find yourself in a social setting, rambling self-righteously about a first-world problem that you think is actually important, only to be interrupted by a witty quip from a friend with the intention of providing perspective?

Suddenly, you're disarmed of your serious-sword and quickly handed a clown horn, all in one moment. That moment, brought to you by the makers of "get over yourself" proves to be an inviting, humility-inducing tonic.

In other words, just what you needed.

The same applies to a yoga practice. Yoga is synonymous with balance, and not just in the physical sense. A healthy hybrid of strength and flexibility, combined with a perspective-inducing formula of diligence and levity, can help us keep balance as the broad stroke that paints our yoga landscape. When you bring it, bring it with a smile.

Hey, it's only yoga.

When first-timers walk into my studio, my staff hands them an introduction sheet to calm their nerves. It is laced with levity because I don't want them to take themselves too seriously. Here's how it reads:

What is about to happen? What just happened? What the #*!*?

No worries! You are not going to die today.

On the contrary, you are about to feel reborn.

Remember that yoga is a diagnostic tool. Throughout the first few weeks of practicing, your body will be sending you messages that may not read like love letters from Ryan Gosling or Penelope Cruz.

These messages may come in the form of dizziness, nausea, soreness and disorientation.

Guess what? That's good news. These are common complaints, and as you adjust to the yoga series and the heat, the symptoms will dissipate and you will start to feel like a superhero—minus the colored tights!

In the meantime, here's how you can help:

- Drink lots of water before and after class. Any water: tap, bottled, spring, Chardonnay. Whatever. Toronto's tap water is the 3rd best in North America, and it actually tastes good, but it's your call.

- Try to stay away from liquids that rhyme with "toffee" or "cruise" before class. Moderation is key in this area. They both dehydrate, making you feel like a fruit fly in a beer keg. Not what you're after.

- Don't eat for a few hours before class and if you do, keep it light; and by "light", we don't mean ordering the wings instead of the ribs.

- Wear less clothing. The truth is, five minutes into class, you could be wearing dental floss and no one would care. Okay, they would, but don't be shy. Less clothing equals more comfort. You. Look. Hot! And it just gets better!

- Let go of the fear. There are many necessary cautions in this life, such as lion-taming, high-rise window cleaning and owning too many Black Sabbath records, but hot yoga is not one of them. It exists to heal you, not hinder you.

Unnecessary worry will just get in the way of your progress. That said, you are the barometer for your body. If you need to take a break because you feel overwhelmed in ANY way, simply sit or lie down. Yoga is NOT about competition or performance. Just try to stay in the room and stay focused.

At BeHot Yoga Toronto, we provide a safe environment with highly-qualified instructors who will accommodate all that encompasses your yoga journey. Always come to us with ANY concerns.

EMBRACE THE THREE R's!

Your body will REACT (not fun), REPAIR (somewhat fun) and then REMODEL (so much fun)! It's not a linear progression, so be patient with yourself and your practice. Some days will suck. Others will enlighten. Simply observe and learn. Try to practice at least three times a week.

Welcome CHANGE and, by all means, have fun. You're doing your body, mind and spirit a great service with this noble commitment to yoga.

Okay, let's do this! Water? Check. Mat? Check. Towel? Check.

Now, check the ego (that silly thing that gets in your way) and let's get hot and healthy.

Sometimes, I like to watch a student's face as they sit down and read the sheet. The smile it produces along with the sudden drop of their shoulders away from their ears is a testament to the fact that lightening the air *a little* can help *a lot*.

Chapter 26

IT'S THE YOGA, STUPID

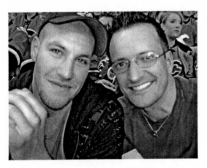

Paul with nephew and NHL hockey
player, Brandon Prust

"They criticize me for harping on the obvious; if all the folks in the United States would do the few simple things they know they ought to do, most of our big problems would take care of themselves."

—Calvin Coolidge

Fitness and health have somehow become one and the same in western culture, and the reality is that while the two appear to create a good hybrid—one complimenting the other— the results of the pairing may just have the same outcome as that of matching up Bonnie and Clyde.

We often traumatize our bodies and joints in the name of fitness and sometimes our intentions are in earnest, but the damage being done can be chronic and quite serious. Health is not present in this picture.

Professional athletes are fit, but are they healthy?

To use just one example, my nephew, Brandon Prust, is a professional hockey player for the Montreal Canadiens. He has enjoyed a successful career, no doubt, but it has come at the price of his body, and arguably, his overall wellness.

His conditioning and level of performance is exemplary—you don't get to the NHL without exceptional skills—and there is no question that he is what would be deemed "fit" in our society.

But, on the road to greatness, Brandon's body has tallied up more bangs than the Red Light District.

The list: Concussion at age 19, broken jaw at 20, hip surgery at 23, another concussion at 24, another broken jaw at 25, shoulder surgery at 27, shoulder separation at age 29, dislocated rib at 29, torn oblique at age 30.

Brandon is strong, resilient and fit, no doubt—at the time of this writing, his career continues, interrupted often by injuries, of course—but his health has been compromised by his passion and dedication to a life as a professional hockey player.

Luckily, it's not too late for Brandon. He can still heal and benefit from yoga by applying his extraordinary work ethic into a regular practice.

More and more athletes are upping their game by including yoga as part of their training regimen. Tennis star

Andy Murray credits Bikram yoga for building his endurance, and athletes from NBA great Lebron James to Toronto Blue Jays baseball player Brett Lawrie praise yoga for increasing their level of mental strength—a valuable performance component for any pro athlete.

That said, not enough is being done by professional sports organizations to make yoga a staple in the workout diet of their athletes, and it could be argued that this is because they are not focused on the big health picture of the individuals they employ. They simply want results at any cost, even the long-term health of a human being. This is why more pro athletes are making the wise, independent choice to include yoga in their lives and plan for a retirement that won't have them picking out wheelchairs.

Too many athletes are enduring painful arthritis and endless surgeries in their early 30s, and the debilitating damage done to their bodies is being provisionally tempered through the quick fix of a cortisone shot or the chronic use of pain pills such as Percocet. Cautionary tales involving overdose and depression due to dependence and lack of helpful resources within their organization are becoming too frequent.

A dark cloud is hovering over many professional athletes, turning pro sports into a dangerous game whose opponent isn't who stands before him, but what lies ahead of him.

While these cases, with pro sports as a backdrop, may seem a little more extreme than others, there are smaller deals—save the notoriety—being made with the devil for the esthetic merits of fitness by millions of others every day.

An addiction to running can do gradual but severe damage to the hip and knee joints, and may not be having the cardio effects one might believe.

In the book *Body by Science*, co-author Dr. McGuff explains—through detailed research—how aerobic training became erroneously linked with cardiovascular fitness, despite the contention that it does little to nothing for the health of the heart. In addition to the development of osteoarthritis of the knees and hips later in life, ultimately requiring joint replacements, he asserts the following:

> The scientific literature is filled with data that strongly make the case that long distance runners are much more likely to develop cardiovascular disease, atrial fibrillation, cancer, liver and gallbladder disorders, muscle damage, kidney dysfunction (renal abnormalities), acute micro thrombosis in the vascular system, brain damage, spinal degeneration and germ-cell cancers than are their less active counterparts.

Dr. McGuff footnotes each of his evaluations.

Yoga does not share such risks.

There are certainly articles out there condemning yoga as a claimed cure-all, but that's because it's not. Nothing is.

But it is important to point out that the main objective of any yoga practice is to move towards—and maintain—optimal health.

Fitness, at best, is a simple by-product.

Trash-talking articles about the "suspected" benefits of yoga are largely laughable because they don't carry any data to back up the sensationalized assertion that yoga does not work.

If I wanted to grab a reader's attention in a society in which millions of people are turning to yoga to help with what ails 'em, as a journalist, the first thing I would do would be to plan an all-out assault on the activity. It makes for interesting, outside-the-box reading. That's just the nature of media these days. To not identify the motive as a business tactic to sell papers or magazines would be as naïve as thinking a pharmaceutical company is only interested in your health.

Or, to sneakily obtain your interest, I would write a book entitled, *I Hate Yoga,* with the sly, backhanded-Buddha motive of actually getting people to try it and love it. Insert wink emoticon here.

So, how do you discern? What's a gimmick and what isn't?

I would start with 5,000 years of history documenting the healing properties of yoga leading up to a quick Google search with these two words: Yoga and benefits. On the first page alone, you'll likely see an article from *The National Geographic* in February 2014, entitled, "New Study Shows Yoga Has Healing Powers"—if it's not trumped by pages of studies that have taken place since.

If that's not enough to twist your brain, go to a local bookstore and pick up *Yoga Anatomy* by Leslie Kaminoff and Amy Matthews, that includes detailed descriptions of each yoga posture and how it affects your physiology.

It was my initial intention in writing this chapter to list numerous studies on the endless benefits of yoga—there are many—but it was also my full intention in writing this book to not completely bore the reader; besides, while I have used data and studies selectively in previous chapters, information in the form of detailed research in our day and age is so easy to come by, it only made sense to give you, the reader, a little homework.

To give you a framework, comprehensive studies include documentation on the health benefits of yoga for: Arthritis, cancer, cognition and quality of life, diabetes, strength and flexibility, asthma, regulating blood pressure, insomnia, joint pain, back ailments, circulation problems and headaches—to name just a few.

More importantly, you will quickly understand that yoga—when practiced responsibly and in moderation—can help you with moving towards (and maintaining) a healthy life.

And when people start to ask you why you look so lucid, vibrant and damn energetic, just look at them with a sly smile and say without a hint of smugness: "It's the yoga, stupid."

Chapter 27

CONVICTED OF KILLING TIME

"Time is what we want most, but what we use worst."
—William Penn

There's a joke I quite enjoy: A mother is sitting with her young son and he says earnestly, "Mom, when I grow up, I want to be a musician," to which the mother replies, "Oh, son. You know you can't do both."

As children, we had no limitations on our dreams. No disclaimers. No reality checks; no monetary expectations to match our heartfelt desires and high-reaching goals.

Try explaining to a child that a "dragon slayer" is not a realistic vision given the tax implications, ineligibility for health insurance and declining job opportunities. A blank stare will follow. You've lost him. Not only that, but you just messed with something very pure: Heartfelt conviction.

I'm going to use my nephew as an example once again because, as our family all watched him grow up, his convictions were clear: Become a professional hockey player. So he did.

Not all stories have this kind of fairy tale tag, but he did not arrive where he is without great difficulty. What allowed his dream to flourish was an uncompromising refusal to negotiate with anything that stood in the way of his convictions.

We are all afforded this choice.

The truth is, as adults, our convictions are often tainted—sometimes very understandably—by the daunting scene of the world before us. But what we see as a "realistic perspective" can often and easily be dismantled as mere excuse. Failing in our convictions is easy and, as stated earlier, it happens; but maintaining them through adversity is what makes the word so powerful and laced with integrity.

I hear excuses disguised in "reality" every day. I am guilty of them myself. I won't list them because my purpose at this point is to inspire, not to chide. That said, the main culprit for absence from the yoga practice appears to be something that, from all I can gather, doesn't really have any true power over conviction. It's called "time."

Conviction can transcend and conquer time. Every. Time.

If you connect with the untainted vision and relentless purpose of the child you once were, you can break down mythical time barriers and renew the heart-led convictions that once had you ascending to beautifully majestic, magical heights.

A regular yoga practice brings great benefits—a simple truth that, when honored, can never be challenged by time.

It will kill time. Literally. Figuratively. Courageously.

It's no contest. Take out your sword of conviction. Prepare to slay the "Time Dragon."

Chapter 28

TURNING A FEW TRICKS

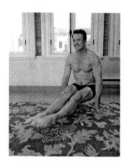

"The most common way people give up their power is by thinking they don't have any."
—Alice Walker

I t's important to understand that the best way to get the most benefits from a yoga practice is to actually practice yoga.

Procrastination is said to be the fear of success, but if you need some motivation to get off your ass and into an asana, here are some tricks you can use that may help.

1) Perspective

How many times have you walked by someone who has been disfigured in an accident, maimed, crippled by disease or handed a physical or mental plight that seems incredibly burdensome, painful and unfair? And how many times have you whispered under your breath: "There but for the grace of God go I?"

Well, I'm here to tell you that I have witnessed a lot of these "less fortunate" people doing yoga. They work with what they have to make sure it operates at an optimal level and here's the kicker: They don't usually see themselves as being "less fortunate" than you.

Yoga brings them closer to who they are regardless of their appearance or ailment.

I had a student with Fibromyalgia, a cruel disorder that limited her breathing and brought with it an incredible amount of pain. She would often have to walk out of the yoga room and take breaks, only to venture back in as soon as she possibly could. She would smile at me through her pain and say over and over again, "It's tough, but the yoga really helps. I'm thankful for it."

She's thankful. How's that for perspective?

My friend and business consultant, Michael Harris, wrote a book entitled, *Falling Down, Getting Up* in which he describes using yoga to help him heal from a childhood accident, vascular surgeries and years of alcohol and drug abuse. It's an inspiring tale of overcoming hardship brought on by a series of unfortunate circumstances and choices.

Yoga played an integral role in his recovery.

When I first started working with Michael, we would connect on Skype and, as is the customary greeting, I would ask him how he's doing.

Each and every time he would exclaim with a genuine smile, "Pretty amazing." And he meant it.

This coming from a man who, given what he's been through, really should not be alive. But he is—and he exudes a happiness and passion so resolute it almost demands an explanation.

If they can take the high road, then so can you.

I know that sounds like a guilt trip, but it's not. It's perspective.

You may not think that yoga can take you to a feel-good level that scales the walls of your current state, but I've seen so many people physically and emotionally enhanced by a yoga practice that not trying it at all seems like its own form of self-neglect.

You may just be missing out on something that not only offers up a personal perspective, but a feeling of clarity that can fill you with gratitude and good fortune.

2) Inspirational quotes

I love inspirational quotations. They feed me and fill me with motivation.

I use my favorites all the time during classes I teach. My students often comment on their potency and how a particular credo gave them a moment of strength or much-needed drive, or took them out of the realm of complacency.

When I doubt my abilities, I conjure up Henry Ford's, "Whether you think you can or whether you think you can't, you're right."

When I feel fear, I break it down into an acronym and turn it into its antonym: False. Evidence. Appearing. Real. (OR) Forgetting. Everything's. All. Right.

When I'm upset about a missed opportunity, I smile as I hear my dad's thick Scottish brogue belting out, "What's for ya, won't go by ya."

When I'm feeling sorry for myself, the perspective-inducing wisdom of Michael J. Fox is quickly used as a cure: "My happiness grows in direct proportion to my acceptance, and in inverse proportion to my expectations."

When I'm feeling commonplace, Dr. Seuss usually has the remedy: "Today you are you. That is truer than true. There is no one on earth who is youer than you."

Pick some quotations that inspire you. Write them down and put them where you'll see them every day—on the fridge, the bathroom mirror and your coffee cup.

Or, if you are apt to do so, get a tattoo. My girlfriend has, "Don't cry because it's over, smile because it happened" written along her spine. I can't count the number of times the visual presence of that quote has put a welcome smile on my face.

No strategy is too cheesy if it lifts your spirits; a well-placed, ringing quotation can become a healing salve for the soul.

3) Leaders

As I said earlier, we don't necessarily need gurus or mentors to help us hit our stride, but we all have individuals we can look up to in proper doses; and we don't necessarily need to be interacting with them personally in order to draw encouragement from their greatness.

For each of us, that figure will be different. But we all likely have a few, and not just of the "what I'd do for an hour with him or her" variety—although there's certainly a place for that as an engine-starter.

No, I'm talking about Mandela, Monet, Hemingway, Gretzky, Obama, Hepburn, Houdini, Ghandi, Streep, Oprah, Chopra, Dickens, Robinson, Mozart, Churchill, Sinatra, Joplin, Lincoln, Keller, Davinci, Atwood, Peron, Disney, Twain, Teresa, Dylan, Warhol and Washington…to name a few.

They all inspire.

Sometimes, we don't just draw from famous people. It's a family member or someone we just met who displays a flash of greatness in front of our own eyes—enough to humble us and take the opportunity to bank the moment for our own use. Whatever works. Just remember there's a difference between idolization and healthy admiration. Be your own guru.

4) Your vision statements

Without splitting the ass of my pants taking bows, I can say with unwavering pride that, as a child, I knew I wanted to act and sing. I didn't know exactly what a life in music theatre would look like. I was a little scared and I've made it clear that I didn't always follow my instincts, but I knew I would be a performer.

Lily Tomlin once said, "When I grow up, I want to be somebody, but now I realize I should have been more specific."

I wish I had been told to write down a vision statement when I was 18 or younger, detailing with precision exactly how I wanted everything to unfold.

It's a powerful exercise.

I do it now for everything. My career. My business. My relationships.

Your vision statements don't have to be made public. They're for you. But you do need them to interact with the energy of the universe, so they need to be put out there. By you. How else can they manifest?

If you don't know what you want, how can it come to fruition?

Make no mistake, it likely will not be a linear path to greatness once you've documented your vision, but where would the fun be in that? Just trust that you have increased your odds considerably.

If you need to be motivated, perhaps the best question to explore would be, "What motivates me?"

So, what motivates YOU?

Sometimes, we need to get out of our own way and grip the reigns of inspiration that have been handed over to us from an outside source. Using tools to motivate us—whether it is an enlightening story, a prophetic quotation, an iconic figure, or an amusing anecdote—is as useful and sensible as using shampoo to clean your hair.

To be our shiny selves, we often need a helping hand.

The strength and accomplishments of others can be our beacon. A potent quotation can be our mood-enhancer. A harrowing story with a triumphant conclusion can be our liberator. A vision statement can be our guide.

Use them in all facets of your life. And use them to get to yoga. Empower yourself by plugging into these outlets whenever and wherever you need.

Being the best you that you can be isn't just good for you—it's good for everyone.

CONCLUSION

"The most difficult thing is the decision to act; the rest is merely tenacity."

—Amelia Earhart

A
t this point, you may suspect that I am actually quite fond of yoga.

Okay, I admit it. I am.

But much like the prodigal son whose return home is curiously celebrated, I can arrive back into the bosom of yoga without judgment. Yoga, after all, does not discriminate and holds out a forgiving hand.

But before my homecoming, I had to abandon yoga, question it, explore its possible misgivings and even hate it.

It's a journey I wanted to take you on with the intention of cathartically bringing you to a place in which you can also have a healthy relationship with yoga—warts and all.

But sometimes, the most effective way to arrive at such a place is to come in through the back door.

I remember seeing the powerful movie, *Capote* with Phillip Seymour Hoffman, in which Truman Capote spends endless hours interviewing a man who took part in the brutal killings of an entire family. Capote was writing the lauded book, *In Cold Blood*, during which time he developed "strong feelings of identification" with the convicted murderer, Perry Smith.

In one scene, someone asks Capote what his endless fascination was with Perry.

His answer is chilling.

"It's as if Perry and I grew up in the same house. And one day, he stood up and went out the back door, while I went out the front."

He saw a slightly altered reflection of himself in Perry Smith. His connection with a man whose fate was determined by darker choices makes me realize how alarmingly fragile and impressionable we are as human beings.

We need help to make the right choices.

I believe yoga is one such choice and I wanted to help you discover it. But, in writing this book, I felt it would be more effective to bring yoga in the back door and whisk everyone in its path out the front.

I think it has that kind of transformational power.

When I'm feeling low, I often sit down at the piano and sing. The songs I choose to bellow out are usually melancholy ballads. Ironically, I slowly begin to hit the other side of the sadness by delving deeper into it.

It's a therapeutic journey that can take place because—however difficult—I am honoring how I feel at that time and facilitating the potential for healing through creative expression.

By exposing my yoga devils and navigating through them with brutal and often blunt candor in this book, I can safely arrive at the conclusion that everything—even yoga—deserves to be carefully dissected and assessed.

Remember, if you can see the Buddha, kill the Buddha.

Each journey we take holds the potential for discovery, but each is also wonderfully subjective. It's *your* journey.

When I was in teacher training, one of our instructors would continuously tell us what we could expect to feel week-to-week. This always got my back up and finally—each time he would dump his formulaic outline on us—I would whisper under my breath, "Fuck you. This is *my* journey."

Whether you're an experienced practitioner, an eager newbie, or a reluctant observer with more than a little curiosity, what happens next is part of *your* journey.

I encourage you to go on your own yoga adventure. Disparagement, frustration and yes, even hate, can be a healthy part of your expedition.

But while embracing those feelings—along the way—it's not only likely that you will gain an astute knowledge of your body, an acceptance of all your so-called flaws, a validation of your unique existence, a friendly relationship with authenticity and an overall strength of body and mind you thought only drugs could induce, but it's also quite possible that you will come to this hearty, smile-inducing conclusion:

I. Love. Yoga.

ABOUT THE AUTHOR

Paul McQuillan is the owner and director of BeHot Yoga Toronto. He has been a yoga teacher for nine years and a professional singer/actor for 30 years. Paul has performed on stages in over 60 cities across North America, including Broadway. He has written several articles for Tonic Magazine and his popular—but controversial—article in Canada's national newspaper, *The Globe and Mail*, entitled "I'm at peace, but I'm not happy about it" was his inspiration for writing *I Hate Yoga*.

He appears in the feature documentary *Planet Yoga* in which his contemporary ideas surrounding yoga are explored.

Paul currently resides in Toronto.

For more information, go to www.paulbmcquillan.com

Speaking Engagements

Paul is currently taking bookings for speaking engagements across North America. If you want to take the fear factor out of yoga and learn how individuals in your company, business or group can benefit by beginning a yoga practice, Paul will take you through an interactive presentation that offers a clear perspective on yoga in today's world and provides you with the motivational tools to get started.

For more information, go to www.paulbmcquillan.com or www.themorganjamesspeakersgroup.com

BeHot Yoga Teacher Training Program

If you wish to become a certified yoga teacher, BeHot Yoga Teacher Training takes place in Toronto each year under the direction of author Paul McQuillan. Dedicated, experienced teachers, health care practitioners and business experts run the program.

To learn more, go to www.behotyogatoronto.com

ACKNOWLEDGEMENTS

The musings presented in this book would not have come to fruition were it not for the definitively etched influences of many remarkable people—all who have been an integral part of my life thus far—giving my thoughts and ideas the space needed to take off. They all laid the foundation for me to conjure up enough courage to speak from my heart, and to be as silly as possible while doing so. Thank you for your respect and love—but mostly, for never letting me take myself too seriously.

To John Salvatore, for showing me that discipline and humor are great bedmates; to Tony Sanchez, for reigniting my passion for yoga by using the tools of wisdom and a walk-the-talk philosophy; to Darren Voros, for always identifying my strengths and weaknesses better than anyone I have ever met, but fully embracing both; to Eddie Glen, for being a joyous, inimitable constant in my life; to Teshia Maher, for your yoga expertise and for showing me that resilience and healing exist in multiple backbends; to Winny Clarke and Olivia Holland, for the genuine smiles and professional integrity you bring to work each day, and for listening to my daily rants at the yoga studio and convincing me that you are actually interested; to David Mucci, whose brilliant mind and innovative spirit always leave me awe-struck; to Alex Mustakas, for fostering my abilities as a performer and providing a platform for creative expression throughout my life; to Lindsey Love for your street-smart advice and sobering honesty; to Peter Johnston for his brilliant mind and gracious spirit; to Pattie Lovett-Reid and Jim Reid for your kindness, and for igniting months of reflection within me following each dinner we share.

To David Hancock and Morgan James Publishing for your unwavering belief in this book; to Michael Harris, my friend and business coach, who taught me very quickly that no superlative is an exaggeration when it comes to my life vision.

To my nephew Brandon, who is the very definition of work-ethic; to my sisters Theresa and Lorraine for their unconditional love, always being my best audience when it comes to my ridiculousness, and for your continuous need to spoil me; to my brother Kevin, whose heart is softer than he will ever let on; to my mother, for showing me by example how much joy is to be found in books and whose first reaction to my news—told over the phone—of having written a book was, "I don't usually drink alone, but tonight I'm having a rum and coke"; to my step-mother, Patricia, whose pure and steady influence in my life has been a beacon of goodness; to my dear late father, who I miss so deeply and whose loss I still cannot bring myself to feel the full depth of—but whose strength, humility, humor and immense love are engrained in the very depths of my being.

To Ashley. Without you, the motivation, encouragement and perspective needed to write this book would not have existed. Thank you for letting me read to you every night for months on end and reflecting passionately and intelligently on the words. You are the smartest, funniest woman I have ever known.

To the yoga students at my studio for providing me with the awareness that continuous learning is not just an option, but a necessity.

All of these distinctive influences have created a melting pot of ideas, opinions, stories and anecdotes within me to draw from; in the words of Oscar Wilde, a man "becomes an echo of someone else's music, an actor of a part that has not been written for him."

Lastly, I would like to thank *you*, the reader, for allowing me to impart the musings—however arguable, loved or hated—of this book upon you.

RESOURCES

BeHot Yoga Toronto,
43 Colborne St.,
Toronto, Ontario, Canada. M5E 1E3
Website: www.behotyogatoronto.com Phone: 416 203 2382
Author website: www.paulbmcquillan.com
Tony Sanchez's website: tonysanchezyoga.com

Helpful and inspirational books:

    Falling Down, Getting Up—Michael Harris

    Hell-Bent—by Benjamin Lorr

    Anatomy of the Spirit—by Carolyn Myss

    Open—by Andre Agassi

    Yoga Anatomy—by Leslie Kaminoff

    Great By Choice—by Jim Collins

    The Power of Now—by Echart Tolle

    Quiet—by Susan Cain

    Body By Science—by John Little and Doug McGruff

REFERENCES

Andre Agassi, *Open* (Vintage Books, 2010)

Susan Cain, *Quiet* (Crown Publishing Group, 2013)

Leslie Kaminoff, *Yoga Anatomy* (Human Kinetics Publishers, 2009)

Benjamin Lorr, *Hell-Bent* (St. Martin's Press, 2012)

John Little and Doug McGuff , Body By Science (McGraw-Hill Professional Publishing, 2008)

Carolyn Myss, *Anatomy Of The Spirit* (Crown Publishing Group, 1997)

Echart Tolle, *The Power of Now* (New World Library, 2004)

Jeffrey A. Kottler, Ph.D, "What Really Leads To Change In People's Lives," Psychology Today, July 24, 2013, http://www.psychologytoday.com/blog/change/201307/what-really-leads-change-in-people-s-lives

"Yoga In America Study 2012," Yoga Journal, 2012, http://
www.yogajournal.com/press/yoga_in_america

"Addiction Recovery: How Yoga Can Help," NCADD, http://
ncadd.org/in-the-news/432-addiction-recovery-how-
yoga-can-help

"Energy Medicine," Wikipedia, accessed on July 10, 2014,
http://en.wikipedia.org/wiki/Energy_medicine

Michele and Robert Root-Bernstein, "Einstein On Creative
Thinking: Music and the Intuitive Art of Scientific
Imagination", Psychology Today, March 31, 2010, http://
www.psychologytoday.com/blog/imagine/201003/
einstein-creative-thinking-music-and-the-intuitive-art-
scientific-imagination

Raj Raghunathan, "How Negative Is Your Mental Chatter,"
Psychology Today, October 10, 2013, http://www.
psychologytoday.com/blog/sapient-nature/201310/how-
negative-is-your-mental-chatter

Oliver Burkeman, "The Power of Negative Thinking," New
York Times, August 4, 2012, http://www.nytimes.
com/2012/08/05/opinion/sunday/the-positive-power-of-
negative-thinking.html?_r=0

"Demographics of Toronto," Wikipedia, accessed on July 10,
2014, http://en.wikipedia.org/wiki/Demographics_of_
Toronto

"Prescription Drug Use Continues to Increase: U.S.
Prescription Drug Data for 2007-2008", CDC—Centres
For Disease Control and Prevention, September 2010,
http://www.cdc.gov/nchs/data/databriefs/db42.htm

"Addressing Prescription Drug Abuse in the United States—Current Activities and Future Opportunities" U.S. Department of Health and Human Services, accessed July 10, 2014, http://www.cdc.gov/HomeandRecreationalSafety/pdf/HHS_Prescription_Drug_Abuse_Report_09.2013.pdf

"Trend Watch: More U.S. Doctors Prescribing Yoga, Meditation," The Independent, May 10, 2011, http://www.independent.co.uk/life-style/health-and-families/trend-watch-more-us-doctors-prescribing-yoga-meditation-2281940.html

Jamie Hale, "Scared Straight? Not Really," Psychcentral, accessed on July 10, 2014, http://psychcentral.com/blog/archives/2010/11/26/scared-straight-not-really/

"Boredom", Wikipedia, accessed on July 10, 2014, http://en.wikipedia.org/wiki/Boredom

Mark Prigg, "Trusting your instincts really does work, say scientists. You'll be right 90% of the time," Daily Mail, November 12, 2012, http://www.dailymail.co.uk/sciencetech/article-2231874/Trusting-instincts-really-does-work-say-scientists.html

"Caroline Myss, Spiritual Author, Explains Why Intuition Is Often a Source Of Suffering," Huffington Post, updated February 20, 2014, http://www.huffingtonpost.com/2014/02/20/caroline-myss-intuition-suffering_n_4818429.html

Susan Brink, "New Study Shows Yoga Has Healing Powers," National Geographic, February 7, 2014, http://news.

nationalgeographic.com/news/2014/02/140207-yoga-cancer-inflammation-stress/

"Controversial Bikram Yoga Guru Likes the Heat", ABC News—Nightline, January 16, 2013, accessed July 17, 2014, http://abcnews.go.com/Nightline/video/controversial-bikram-yoga-guru-likes-heat-18234510

Rachel Maclean, "Shortened songs at AMP Calgary radio station draw polarized feelings", CBC News, updated Aug. 7, 2014, http://www.cbc.ca/news/canada/calgary/short-songs-at-amp-calgary-radio-station-draw-polarized-feelings-1.2730364

Loraine Despres, "Yoga's Bad Boy: Bikram Choudhury" Yoga Journal, accessed August 10, 2014, http://www.yogajournal.com/lifestyle/328

CPSIA information can be obtained at www.ICGtesting.com
Printed in the USA
BVOW02s0647181114

375597BV00005B/97/P